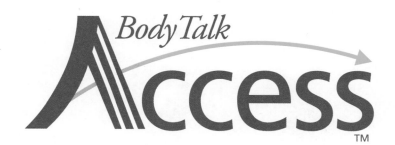

BodyTalk Access

A new path to family and community health

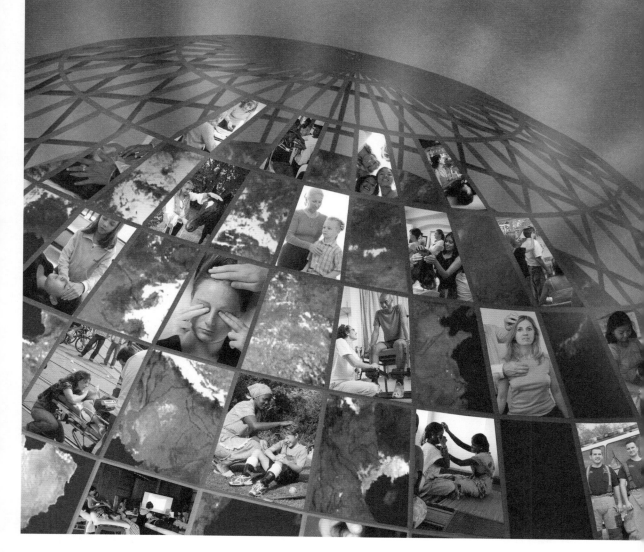

BodyTalk Access

A new path to family and community health

by John Veltheim, D.C., B.Ac.
Published by the International BodyTalk Association

First published in May 2008

By the International BodyTalk Association

2750 Stickney Point Road, Suite 203

Sarasota, FL 34231

ISBN 978-1-929762-16-3

Printed in the USA

Also by John Veltheim

The BodyTalk System

Published by PaRama

Email: office@bodytalksystem.com

Web sites:

www.ibaglobalhealing.com

www.bodytalkaccess.com

www.bodytalkfoundation.org

TABLE OF CONTENTS

FOREWORD

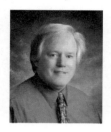

"Small is powerful" is a fundamental principle of energy medicine. The expression perfectly describes this little book. The short time you spend reading *BodyTalk Access: A new path to family and community health* may change your life. John Veltheim has spent many years accumulating a vast knowledge and wisdom about the human body, and has taught his revolutionary techniques around the world. Now he has distilled his remarkable insights into a simple and straightforward summary that will show you what BodyTalk is and what it means for millions of people in every part of the Earth.

In a time when new energy techniques are being developed almost daily, BodyTalk stands out as perhaps the easiest and yet most powerful method you can learn. This applies to everyone, whether you are a medical doctor, an athlete, a mother, a kindergarten student, a therapist of any kind or a Ph.D. candidate. The methods described here will expand your world by enabling you and those around you to experience healthier and happier lives. Try these techniques and see what happens!

BodyTalk Access describes a deceptively simple process that is urgently needed in all of the developed nations, where healthcare systems are not only failing but are simultaneously pushing toward economic collapse. Access is equally important for Third World nations that are entirely lacking in a medical infrastructure - for places where the closest emergency medical care may be many miles away, with no other transportation than walking. John Veltheim has a generosity of spirit that has compelled him to form the International BodyTalk Foundation that is giving this teaching to many impoverished peoples around the world.

I have met BodyTalk practitioners in many places, from New Zealand to Germany to California to England and so on, and they are all eager and delighted to be able to offer BodyTalk to anyone who needs it. Why are they so excited? For many it is because a short course lasting only a few hours has given them powerful tools that they can use with confidence on their families and friends when sickness or injury or medical emergency threatens health and happiness. Many have gone on to make BodyTalk a highly rewarding profession. It is a delight to see this book in print!

James L. Oschman, Ph.D., author of *Energy Medicine: the scientific basis* and *Energy Medicine in Therapeutics and Human Performance.*

Dr. Oschman presenting a keynote seminar during the 2007 IBA Members Conference in Clearwater Beach, Florida, USA

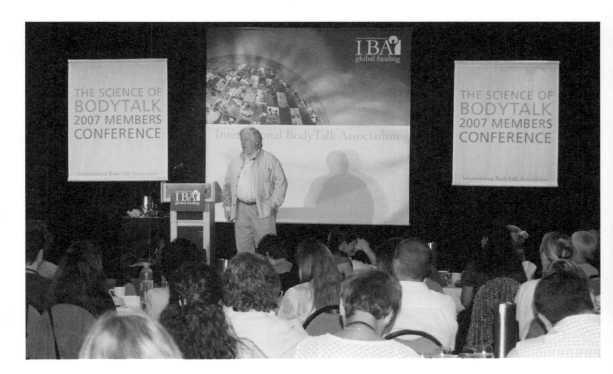

ABOUT THE AUTHOR

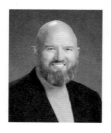

Dr. John Veltheim is a chiropractor, traditional acupuncturist, philosopher and teacher. In 1995, he developed The BodyTalk System™, a revolutionary healthcare regimen that utilizes state-of-the-art energy medicine to optimize the body's internal communications and allows it to more effectively respond to injury and illness. The System and its related wellness and personal growth programs draw on natural energy fields to bring stability, well-being and balance to people, animals and the environment.

Born in Australia, John was a martial arts instructor for 10 years and has a long history of involvement in human potential studies. John, who has served as a board member for the Chiropractic, Naturopathic and Acupuncture professions in Australia, also wrote the curriculum and served as Principal for the Brisbane College of Acupuncture and Natural Therapies for five years. In addition, he was Chairman of the Federation of Australian Acupuncture Colleges.

His extensive post-graduate studies have included applied kinesiology, bioenergetic psychology, osteopathy, sports medicine, counseling, comparative philosophy and theology. John has written several books on the topics of acupuncture, Reiki and BodyTalk. He has specialized in incorporating dynamical systems theory into the medical model and energy medicine in particular.

John and his wife Esther (author of *Beyond Concepts: the investigation of who you are not* and *Who Am I?: the seeker's guide to nowhere*) have been lecturing internationally for nearly 20 years. They currently live in Sarasota, Florida, where they founded the International BodyTalk Association.

MY GOAL IN BODYTALK ACCESS IS TO MAKE THESE SIMPLE TOOLS AVAILABLE TO INDIVIDUALS, SO THEY CAN USE THEM TO HELP MAINTAIN THE HEALTH OF THEIR FAMILIES AND COMMUNITIES.

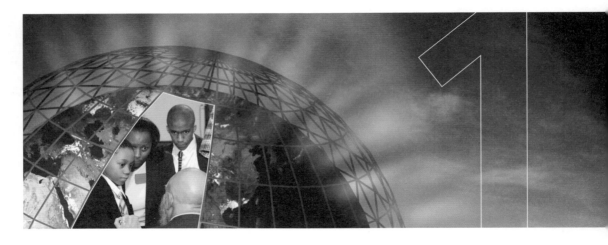

Chapter 1 A Brief History of BodyTalk

BODYTALK ORIGINATED MAINLY OUT OF PERSONAL NECESSITY.

Epstein-Barr Virus (EBV) is a common human virus that causes infectious mononucleosis and plays a role in the emergence of two rare forms of cancer: Burkitt's lymphoma and nasopharyngeal carcinoma.

After many years in a high-volume clinic in Brisbane, Australia, practicing acupuncture, Chinese medicine, chiropractic and naturopathy, my own health caught up with me. As a result of the long hours I kept in practice, as well as my duties running a college and serving as one of its senior lecturers, my health declined. Ultimately, I was diagnosed as having a very serious illness, a very bad strain of the **Epstein Barr virus**, and even was told that I might not live, as it had done extensive damage to my liver.

I originally treated the virus with acupuncture and Chinese herbs, and the illness went from an acute to a chronic stage, manifesting primarily in severe chronic fatigue that nothing seemed to change. I subsequently spent many years with a body temperature over 100 degrees and with constant pain, cramping and extreme fatigue.

I tried everything, and contacted everyone I knew. I used acupuncture and herbs, fasting and diets. I traveled around the world seeking the best practitioners I could find, but nothing seemed to help.

At this stage I had actually sold my clinic and was living a much quieter life on the lecture circuit teaching philosophy, Reiki and various aspects of stress management. Eventually I found myself in New Zealand, where I encountered **Dr. Tracy Livingston**, an osteopath and acupuncturist who had taken some training sessions with me and knew of my illness. She told me that she and some colleagues were investigating the idea of stimulating the body's immune response to chronic viruses and asked if she could treat me using this method.

It was quite a "way-out" idea she proposed, loosely based on applied kinesiology (AK) principles with which I was familiar as a former AK teacher. So I agreed to allow her to do the work.

To start the treatment, Dr. Livingston took a small drop of my blood and put it on a tissue in my navel, which, I knew was a very high-energy center from which the body could register vibrations. Then she started a tapping process on my head.

That was it. Three days later, I was clear of the virus, and it was a completely new beginning for me.

I was very excited about the result and went back and asked for more details. She told me that this was totally new work that seemed to have startling effects and asked me to look into it.

So I did research and examined the technique and found that what they had happened upon utilized a very important principle from a clinical point of view; that is, working through the energy circuits in the body and being able to access the underlying energy blueprint.

"I spent many years constantly searching for something that fulfilled my overwhelming urge to help myself and others with their physical and mental wellbeing. When John developed and taught BodyTalk it made perfect sense to me as it built on the work I was already doing and gave me more applications and power to my treatments, plus a solid theoretical philosophy that dovetailed with original osteopathic philosophy."
- Dr. Tracy Livingston

Using blood (or, as I later found out, saliva) as a signal carrier and activating the brain causes the immune system to launch an assault on any chronic virus, infection or parasite.

Although I was extremely excited about the technique, I was very reluctant to get heavily involved, because I had vowed never to get back into mainstream healthcare. However, my wife, Esther, and I decided that this was far too important to let go. We knew that, particularly in Western developed countries, chronic fatigue in different forms, whether it be chronic viruses, chronic parasites or chronic allergies, strikes around one in five persons and was one of the major illnesses that often could not be treated successfully by either traditional or alternative medicine.

Thus I decided that I would spend time investigating and developing this principle further. Eventually, I found many applications for it, using my background in various alternative therapies. I then developed a list of techniques that, when applied, seemed to get tremendous results in a variety of diseases. These techniques became the first BodyTalk seminar.

At this stage, the major emphasis of BodyTalk was the treatment of chronic disorders. By further utilization of the techniques, however, I was able to address quite a large spectrum of diseases, particularly digestive, endocrine, emotional and stress-related conditions.

I started teaching BodyTalk in 1995. I first taught the system in Malta and England, and then in Australia and New Zealand. It caught on quite quickly as people found they were getting very good results with this simple approach.

Though it was probably more correctly categorized as a sophisticated form of energy medicine, we were describing the system as "acupuncture without needles." At the same time, we were aware it was getting results that actually could not be achieved with acupuncture, much less other alternative or drug therapies.

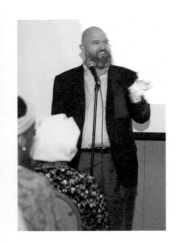

Public Lecture in Chicago, Illinois USA in 2005.

There were two streams of development of the BodyTalk System. One focused on the practical techniques and the creation of protocols and procedures for using them. The other dealt with the philosophical basis; that is, the understanding behind what we were doing. Esther and I developed those streams as a team. Esther focused on the philosophical and psychological input, and I concentrated on the physical application in practice. Over the years, this process has continued.

By 1998, I had been teaching for quite a long time, but I realized that if I wanted to develop BodyTalk further, I had to go back into practice – despite my earlier reluctance. I ended up in Sarasota, Florida, working in a clinic with an acupuncturist. I deliberately did not sit for licensing in the United States because I knew that if I came across any tough cases, I would be tempted to fall back on chiropractic, acupuncture, homeopathy or other disciplines I had learned. Instead, I practiced as a layperson, and this made sure that all I could use was BodyTalk.

Things progressed very quickly after that. Within 90 days, there was a 12-month waiting list in my practice, all because of the results I was getting. During that period of practice, I was able to develop the techniques and perfect the procedures and protocols to a point that I had a system that could be taught to anybody and garner immediate results. I started teaching seminars and also started training some of my top students to be instructors.

During the next few years, BodyTalk developed dramatically. As this is being written in 2008, BodyTalk is being taught in more than 30 countries in eight languages. Our headquarters remain in Sarasota, Florida, but we also have a European branch, near Kempton, Germany, and an Australasian branch in Brisbane, Australia.

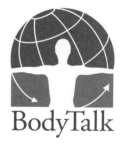

As of 2008, there are nearly 1500 Certified BodyTalk Practitioners in 33 countries around the globe.

To locate one nearest you, visit the official website at www.bodytalksystem.com

It has been an exciting period of growth for BodyTalk. Not only have we taught many thousands of people to use BodyTalk, we now have more than 100 instructors and are branching into many different areas.

BodyTalk continues to be dynamic. There are always new developments and applications of the basic techniques and, by bringing in some advanced concepts of physics and mathematics, we have been able to streamline the techniques to cover a much wider variety of conditions.

I would point out that BodyTalk never claims to treat diseases *per se*. Rather, the emphasis is on addressing the underlying factors of disease and maintaining the health of the body. One of the main philosophies of BodyTalk is that if the body is functioning well – that is, all the lines of communication are there and all the organs are communicating and operating at their optimum level – then the body itself can maintain health or facilitate the self-healing of day-to-day ailments. Obviously there are limitations to this, such as with serious illnesses or injuries that require drug therapy, surgery and all the other modern medical miracles.

At this point in the ongoing evolution of BodyTalk, the system is branching into specialties. We now find the techniques being used in midwifery, sports medicine, rehabilitation, addiction and, of course, our many practitioners are using BodyTalk in their clinics daily to address the day-to-day ailments of their clients.

It also is fascinating to see that BodyTalk works well on animals and plants, as well as people. Like their parent, BodyTalk, these specialties also are expanding quickly, based on the incredible results attained.

Fast Aid for Severe Injury to Thumb

Karen Fair, CBP - Cape Town, South Africa

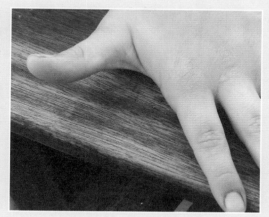

One Friday after school, my son Dane, aged 8 and a scientist in the making, decided to find out how my blender works. He flipped the switch and got his thumb in the way, losing most of the pad of the thumb in the process. My husband was first on the scene and grabbed a white tea towel in an attempt to mop up the blood. The injury was so severe, the towel was drenched in blood by the time I got there.

Dane went into shock and began vomiting. I immediately began applying the BodyTalk Access Fast Aid technique and tapped him consistently as we bundled him into the car for the hospital. The doctor was unable to stitch the wound as there was, quite literally, nothing to stitch together. Instead he cleaned the wound, applied "plastic skin" and bound the thumb in a bandage. All the time, Dane was demanding, "Keep tapping, Mummy!" The startled doctor thought he was asking for water and kept plying him with glass after glass! I must have tapped him a hundred times that day.

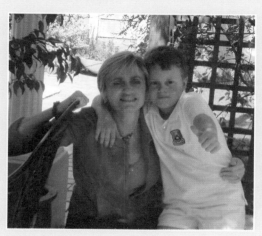

A week later, we returned to the doctor to have the thumb attended to. When he removed the dressing, there was a surprise in store: The pad of the thumb had grown back together again so successfully, the doctor simply cleaned it again and applied a plaster. About two weeks after the episode, there was just a slight pink scar, almost as if drawn in by pen; less than a month later, there is no scar in sight. Dane cannot, in fact, remember which thumb was "blended"!

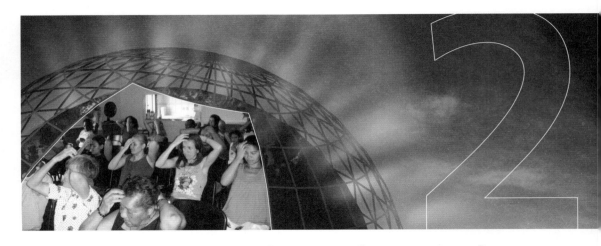

Chapter 2 — The Development of BodyTalk Access

Throughout my many years in the practice and study of healthcare and philosophy, I have formulated certain ideas about the way we should operate in the world from the perspective of wellbeing. As a result, I always have looked for ways of empowering people to rely less on the medical systems and to take more personal responsibility, using sound guidance and principles to look after themselves and their families.

Obviously my background in naturopathy had a lot to do with that, as far as eating right, living right and keeping the mind exercised. However, I wanted to go further. I wanted to empower people even more; I wanted them to be able to treat day-to-day conditions without constant reliance on, and visits to, professional medical care.

While this has been a goal all my professional life, I had never really achieved it in the way in which I wanted. I studied all sorts of simplistic systems, and I usually found that the results were not as good as I wanted. Most of the one-day programs, such as you see with certain cranial work, reflexology or acupressure, did show some results but not what I call professional results. To me, professional results are achieved when you are getting results 70-80 percent of the time. Many self-help treatments tend to make some difference, but they are not totally reliable.

Over the years I became quite despondent about this and found myself focusing on getting good results in my own practice using my current knowledge. Then BodyTalk came along and, when I first developed it, I thought this could create a situation in which we could encourage laypersons to learn the BodyTalk System and help themselves.

THE GOOD NEWS ABOUT THE PROTOCOL AND PROCEDURES OF BODYTALK IS THAT THEY ARE PERFECTLY SAFE

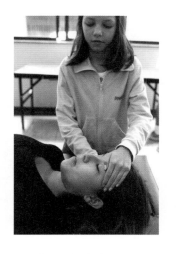

There is nothing they can do to harm people, and in the many years that BodyTalk has been practiced, there are no known cases of harmful side effects, only the occasional temporary fever or gastric activity - signs that the body is fighting off its ailment. So, as it is a completely safe system and, in its early stages, a fairly simple one, I finally thought I would be able to achieve my goal of self empowerment for families and communities.

Quickly, however, I found that to cover the widest variety of ailments, the BodyTalk System had to become reasonably complex, even in the early modules – what we call Modules 1 and 2, which is a four-day intensive program that involves a lot of study and a lot of dedication. And while we have opened it up for laypersons to learn, we found that if they went to all the trouble of learning those modules, they usually went on to become professional BodyTalk practitioners. The advanced levels of BodyTalk are quite sophisticated and require quite a lot of study and knowledge of anatomy, physiology and a large number of other principles around energy medicine.

Access techniques are simple enough that even young children can learn and apply them on friends and family.

So the BodyTalk System over the next several years continued to develop into a whole series of modules that could be quite complex and mainly suitable for people who wanted to be certified BodyTalk practitioners or healthcare providers who wanted to expand their scope of practice and speed up their results.

Energy Medicine vs. Energy Healing

History has documented many people who seem to have been born natural energy healers or spiritual healers. Their results demonstrate significant abilities in bringing about profound changes in the health of the body. One of the drawbacks is that these gifted people can rarely pass on this ability to others at will. The term "energy medicine" is used to refer to energy healing systems that are based on sound scientific and philosophical principles and can be taught to anyone with a desire to use them. In this way they become a useful part of the healing sciences, offering an alternative to the more widely known methods of Western medicine. BodyTalk is such an energy medicine system.

But then things came full circle, and I began to realize that the whole BodyTalk matrix had grown to the point that we could seriously look at the simpler techniques of BodyTalk as being standalone procedures that work extremely well and are easy to learn.

In fact, I came to realize that there were five basic techniques in BodyTalk that could be taught in a short course and could profoundly affect a very wide range of health challenges, as well as serve as an excellent way of maintaining health and optimizing the function of the body.

So I looked into the concept of being able to teach a very simple course over six hours in one day or even two evenings, which would give anyone the ability to address a wide variety of illnesses or injuries that come up on a day-to-day basis. With the help of Sylvia Muiznieks, one of the BodyTalk System's senior instructors, these five BodyTalk techniques were combined and developed into just such a one-day course that anyone can learn.

THE RESULT WAS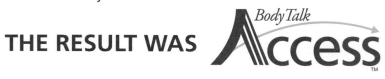

Once I started researching this powerful concept, then put it into practice and saw the results, I realized it was a powerful tool indeed. I came to realize that once people are trained in Access, they are able to maintain the health of their family and friends to an extent where they can dramatically cut down their families' and communities' susceptibility to disease by having the immune system and other body dynamics functioning at their best. Further, we found that the BodyTalk Access program can take care of around 50 to 60 percent of the health challenges that will come up on an average monthly basis.

This was very exciting because it is something that is needed around the globe. This is true whether we are talking of developing nations with little access to healthcare or well-developed countries, where healthcare costs can be extraordinary, requiring a "poor" person to sell his or her home to afford major surgery or to forego meals in favor of costly medication.

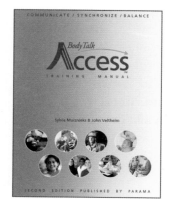

The BodyTalk Access training manual currently is translated and taught in Spanish, English, German, Italian, Swedish, Japanese, Chinese and Portuguese.

My goal in BodyTalk Access is to make these simple tools available to individuals, so they can use them to help maintain the health of their families and communities.

A typical scenario that comes to mind is one of the key factors that helped me to make the decision to go ahead with the Access program. I was on the south side of Chicago, where I had a pilot program treating children with learning disorders using BodyTalk. I was talking to a few of the parents there. I remember one woman, a young, single mother with two children, who pointed out that her income was extremely low, on the order of $10,000 a year, and she did not get sick pay or holiday pay because hers was a "casual" job, that is, one that did not require the payment of benefits by the employer. She had the dilemma that, when her son woke up with a fever or was sick or lethargic, she had to choose between taking him to a clinic and going to work.

The fact was that if she took him to a clinic, she would have to take a day off without pay, which meant that her family would have to go without food since she could not afford both. The reality was that when she took her son to the clinic, her minimum wait was eight hours, and she often waited 12-16 hours for him to be seen. The first time he was treated, he would be seen only by a nurse, who often would give the child three aspirin and tell the mother that, if he was still sick in two days, to come back and they would arrange for him to see a doctor. That, apparently, was the standard procedure.

To me, it was horrific that something like this could happen in a well-developed country such as the United States. I knew we had to do a lot better, and Access could further that goal.

For example, in cities such as Chicago, we train people in the community through the churches or other organizations. This means that this same single mother can now go to a clinic at the local church and quickly receive the Access techniques, which take around six minutes to administer and produce quick results. The great thing about Access is that if it is going to work, it works quickly, with ailments such as viruses and infections turning around in a day or so.

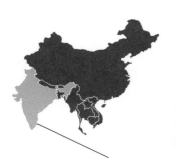

Women in Tamil Nadu, India, practice the BodyTalk Access techniques on each other.

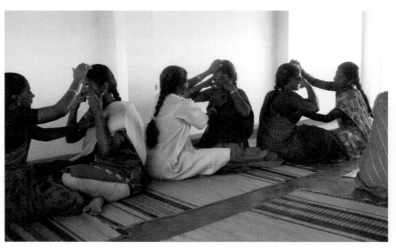

A pictorial version of the Access Manual is available for Instructors. This allows the course to be taught to anyone no matter their language.

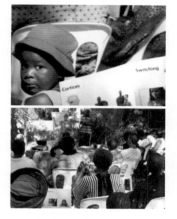

Residents in Botswana, Africa, use the Access pictorial to learn the system.

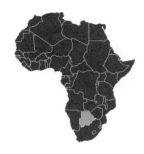

Of course, for a serious complaint, the woman would need to take her son to the hospital for conventional medical care. However, we are finding that, in the small communities where we have set this up, Access is taking care of the majority of the health issues. You can imagine the savings in the community and the savings even for the government.

Consider: If we can get members of the public and local communities taking care of the majority of their healthcare needs for free – just by using very simple, non-invasive techniques – then there will be billions of dollars in savings for countries, whether Third World or highly developed, because healthcare is a huge expense in any country and for any community.

Our goal originally was to arrive at a situation in which every household had someone trained in Access. This, of course, is an ideal, but what a wonderful thing it would be. More recently, we have focused on developing countries, and we now have programs in South Africa, Botswana, Zimbabwe, Kenya, India, Mexico, Brazil and many other less affluent nations, where we are training people as a community. For example, we have villages in South Africa where local community social workers are being taught the BodyTalk Access system. This program is being subsidized by the Access teachers' offering their services for free. Sometimes there are contributions from local governments or philanthropists.

But, one way or the other, we are getting people together for a day, training them and making them confident in using BodyTalk Access. Then those people are going on to look after local residents and make a significant positive change in the general health of the overall community. This is particularly important in areas in which income is miniscule and medical care can be a 20-mile or longer walk away. With most healthcare issues handled easily at home, that income and journey can be reserved for those rare occasions of serious injury or illness.

Needless to say, we are getting tremendous support, not only from the communities, but also from the local governments in these countries, because they see it as a huge cost savings to them. Now they can use the skills of their highly trained doctors and costly equipment in ways that make the most impact, while Access takes care of day-to-day health problems.

The idea is catching on very quickly, and Access is growing extremely fast throughout these countries. That is due to its powerful combination of cost-effectiveness for the governments and local councils, as well as its effectiveness in getting results in a short time.

Access for Cuts from Broken Glass
Shenaaz Khan, CBP - KwaZulu Natal, South Africa

My 11-year-old son went to the shop to buy Coca Cola. He had two 1.25-liter bottles in a carrier bag, which he was transporting on his scooter (the kind you push and go with one leg). He tripped in the road and dropped the glass bottles, which broke. He fell on the glass, cutting himself on his hand by the thumb and on his knee. My hubby and I heard the fall and ran to his aid. He was bleeding so much, we put him in the bathtub. While my hubby was washing the wounds, I was doing Access. The bleeding slowed down and then stopped completely. I was so excited.

My son needed stitches but all the doctors' offices were closed, as it was a Sunday afternoon. So I just kept on doing Access for two or three more times and bandaged him up. Two days later, his hand was still swollen. I did Access to the little pus it still had. Though I did not take my son to the doctor nor give him an antibiotic, about 1-1/2 weeks later, everything had healed nicely.

22

Child's Eczema Gone in Australia

Rosilyn Kinnersley, CBI - Melbourne, Australia

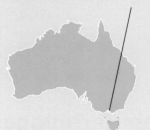

A mother and grandmother took an Access seminar with me together to help their almost 3-year-old son/grandson with severe eczema. They chose to conduct the Access program on the lad three times a day for the 13 days before I could see him for a BodyTalk treatment. By the time he arrived for the BodyTalk session, only two very small red spots remained on his body to show that this child had ever had eczema. His skin was the clearest it had been since he was 3 months old. Access had done a wonderful job of sorting out his eczema condition, which covered 95 percent of his body most of the time.

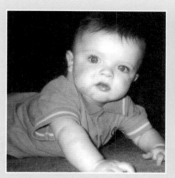 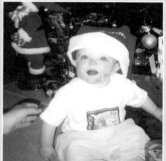

After three further BodyTalk sessions, the little lad is finally a happy and contented boy who loves his bath – after screaming constantly during bath time in agony of the stinging; and he is reveling in playing outdoors in the sun and making mud pies!

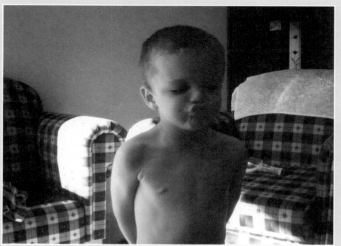

Mum and grandmum are obviously absolutely thrilled and now ready to apply Access to the rest of the family to see what else can change!

Eczema is a chronic, recurring and intensely itchy form of dermatitis, or inflammation of the upper layers of the skin. In Greek, eczema means to" boil over" and this refers to the weeping stage of acute eczema.

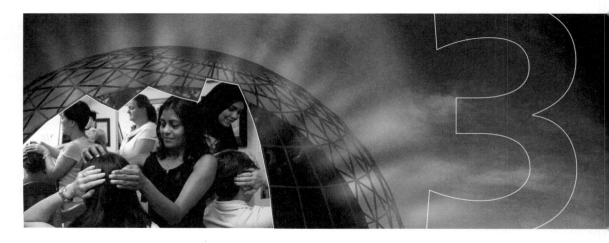

Chapter 3 BodyTalk Access Techniques

BodyTalk Access is a complete system in its own right and stands alone from the general BodyTalk System.

Access comprises five basic techniques – Cortices, Switching, Hydration, Body Chemistry and Reciprocals – that we categorize into two groups.

The first four techniques (Cortices, Switching, Hydration and Body Chemistry) make up Group One and, for full effectiveness, should be done together. They can be applied in just a few minutes as they are very simple techniques.

The fifth technique (Reciprocals) is just a bit more time-consuming; although it also is very simple, it involves the linking up of many different parts of the body. Thus, it is not always part of the original formula. Reciprocals has a very special purpose in first aid and balancing for musculoskeletal problems and can be done separately from the first four.

In this chapter, I will give you a brief explanation of the theory behind each of techniques and why they are part of the system. I also will teach you the first technique, Cortices, in detail so that you can actually try it yourself on family and friends to see just how effective it really is.

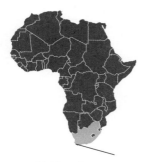

Children in Hout Bay, Cape Town, South Africa walked an average of 1.5 km to the Hout Bay Community Cultural Centre to attend a BodyTalk Access training course.

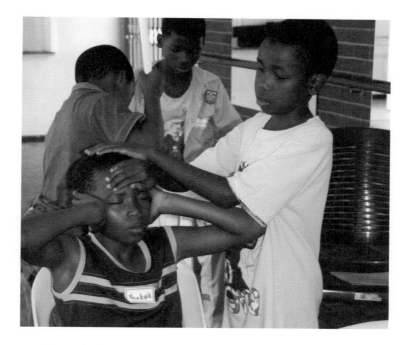

Though these techniques are only a small part of the BodyTalk System, they are probably some of the most significant techniques used in BodyTalk because of their extreme importance in establishing and helping to maintain general health in the body.

Cortices

This is by far the most commonly used technique in BodyTalk. It is the first technique a practitioner will use in almost every treatment, because it is so important in establishing the general healthy functioning of the brain.

A main goal of BodyTalk is to have the brain functioning extremely well, because, when the brain is functioning well, it can control the health of the body by ensuring the right communications are happening and the right instructions are going out.

25

One of the problems in our society is that most peoples' brains are not working well, certainly nowhere near as well as they could. Essentially they have been hijacked by the amygdala system, which is the fight-flight system that is designed to keep us alive.

These days, the stresses of living often cause the amygdala to malfunction.

The brain was originally set up to be very good at handling sudden extreme situations, such as being approached by a wild animal, in which the body had to consider scenarios of either confronting the danger or running from it – hence the fight-flight concept. In those cases, you either fought and won or lost, or you ran and escaped up a tree, into the water or back to home or campfire, away from danger where you could relax again.

However, what is happening in the high-stress world of today is that we are not generally faced with tigers but, rather, with a constant barrage of threats that our body interprets as life-threatening in many ways. These threats are the ordinary stresses of life, such as dealing with financial situations, personal relationships and work pressures; the stress of just driving to and from work and trying to stay alive on the roads, and pollutants and toxins in the food we eat. These are all major stress factors that the average person struggles with daily.

It should be noted that the amygdala is also responsible for the primary survival drives for food, water and sex. When the amygdala complex is disturbed, unhealthy changes will occur with these basic instincts.

Even worse, these stresses affect us even before we are born.

During a pregnancy, the average mother and father can find themselves under a great deal of stress, and this profoundly affects the development of the brain in the fetus. We are finding that more babies are being born with malfunctioning and over-stressed immune and amygdala systems. This leads to a general weakness of the immune system, increasing its susceptibility to infections, viruses and parasites that are difficult to overcome and often remain in a chronic form.

We also are seeing this manifest in the development of allergies to just about everything, from food to environmental factors, in all different levels and in all different stages. In fact, many people can have allergies and not be aware of them because they have no classic allergy symptoms, such as a runny nose or sore eyes. They do not realize that they may have a food allergy that is causing their headaches, pain, Irritable Bowel Syndrome, backache or emotional stress.

Access for a Rash

Sandy Smith - Markham, Ontario, Canada

Molluscum contagiosum is a disease caused by a poxvirus of the Molluscipox virus genus that produces a benign self-limited papular eruption of multiple umbilicated cutaneous tumors. This common viral disease is confined to the skin and mucous membranes.

My youngest son, Tyler, was diagnosed with a rash called "molluscum," which sounds like something from the ocean. Actually, it's a relatively common viral infection of the skin that most often affects children. I was told by doctors that it takes one to two years to go away on its own and they do not treat it.

So for one week I did all the Access techniques with Ty, focusing on the Body Chemistry technique, and now (four weeks later), the rash has almost completely disappeared. The bumps looked like warts growing on top of warts and had been spreading all down the right side of his body. So I was thrilled with the results and had to cancel the appointment with the specialist because there is nothing for her to see anymore.

Either way, we have found that the brain in the average person is far too stressed and has such poor communication it cannot do its job properly. We are seeing this more and more in the youth of today with Attention Deficit Disorder, behavioral problems and major stress disorders. It is alarming how many children are put on Prozac, sedatives, Ritalin and antipsychotics, when really they are just dealing with brains that cannot handle their environment.

The corpus callosum, consisting of over 200 million nerve fibers, is the largest connective pathway in the brain. It connects the left and right sides (hemispheres) to each other.

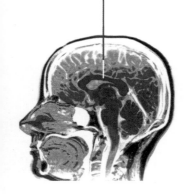

The original Cortices technique is designed to bring about systematic corrections to the brain. The theory is that we are balancing the two halves of the brain, the right and left hemispheres, the masculine and feminine brain, the creative side and the mechanical side.

For most people today, there is a strong masculine-feminine war going on. We call it the battle of the sexes out in the world that we see. However, this battle actually is going on inside the brain between the two value systems or the two ways of dealing with things, such as left-brain logical thinking vs. right-brain intuitive thinking. The fact is, in a healthy person, there is good communication between these extremely important systems, so both ways of thinking can be utilized.

The Cortices technique fosters better communication between the two hemispheres through the **corpus callosum,** thus enabling this communication to occur at all levels.

It is important to reiterate that the BodyTalk System is an energy-based technique, based on the scientific premise that energy comes first and matter follows. It also is important to understand that the latest research in neurosciences has indicated that the actual neurological synaptic transmission of communication between parts of the brain accounts for only some of the communication. A great deal of communication within the brain and from the brain to the rest of the body is occurring at a much higher level through energy systems such as meridians, the flow of electrons, protons, solitons, and electromagnetic frequencies.

The brain and the heart are huge electromagnetic generators, and their frequencies are part of the communication system. When we balance the energic level of the **electromagnetic blueprint**, we are going to profoundly affect all these electrical circuits. Further, we find that, clinically, the balance even affects the physical neurological circuits. The result of this better communication in the brain enables the brain to settle down and better coordinate its activities.

It is well documented that living things such as plants, animals and humans have energy blueprints that are electromagnetic in nature. These blueprints act like the underlying structural and functional matrix of the body and profoundly influence the form and physiology. Science stipulates: "Energy moves first – matter follows." Hence, energy medicine systems such as BodyTalk often focus on changing the blueprint to bring about lasting changes in structure and function.

The Cortices technique also improves circulation within the brain – on many levels. Besides the obviously important blood circulation within the brain, the circulation of the cerebrospinal fluid and the lymphatic drainage of waste-product electrolytes from brain activity also are increased. In addition, the flow of meridian energy and other subtle energy systems critical for healthy brain function are improved. Each time we perform the Cortices treatment, we are improving the total circulation systems. If we perform this technique regularly, we will see continued improvement in the function of the brain.

Shock is a serious, life-threatening medical condition in which insufficient blood flow reaches the body tissues. As the blood carries oxygen and nutrients around the body, reduced flow hinders the delivery of these components to the tissues and can stop the tissues from functioning properly.

The other aspect of the Cortices treatment came from my own clinical observations. We found that when we use the Cortices treatment for people who are in **shock**, it has a miraculous ability to bring them out of that state. For example, we have paramedics who attend to car accidents and see people walking around in a daze. We know from a medical point of view that when the body is in a state of shock, it does not look after the internal mechanisms of the body well at all. Therefore, if that accident victim was internally hemorrhaging in the lungs or in the bowel while in the state of shock, the hemorrhaging would not be controlled.

When we bring them out of shock with the Cortices technique, the body will start to respond and shut down internal hemorrhages. It has been shown that some people who die from accidents and traumas actually die because their bodies were not able to come out of shock early enough for repair to occur. This is why bringing a person out of shock is very important but, from a medical point of view, hard to do. From clinical experience, however, we know that paramedics who have used the Cortices treatment have helped victims almost instantly come out of shock. There have even been cases in which someone was openly bleeding through the skin or experiencing an arterial bleed, and the bleeding stopped as a result of tapping out the Cortices.

Coma Phenomenon 1
Anne Baguhn, CBP - Hamburg, Germany

Several years ago, I took my first BodyTalk class with Dr. Marita Kufe in Hanover, Germany. When I returned to my home in Hamburg, I right away decided I must try to use some of the BodyTalk techniques that I had just learned on my patients. (I am an occupational therapist and was working at the time in a coma ward at a hospital in Hamburg - Bramfeld.) I didn't know quite where to begin, so I decided to do only the Cortices technique on 10 of the patients. I then went home at the end of my shift. The next day when I arrived back, there was a terrific commotion because six patients had awakened from their comas! These were diabetes patients and accident victims, some of whom had been in comas for many months. They still had diabetes and they still needed a great deal of recovery from their injuries – but they came out of their comas and were immediately transferred off my wing for further treatment.

Coma Phenomenon 2
Marci Hettich - Minot, North Dakota, USA

I had finished my first BodyTalk class and wanted more "proof" that BodyTalk works. I had read about the German nurse whose coma patients had regained consciousness after receiving Cortices, so I decided to do the technique on the coma patients I see in the ICU at the hospital where I work as an occupational therapist. Over the next seven months, I did Cortices on ten coma patients, and nine of them regained consciousness that same day or the next.

The results have been so amazing that I continue to do Cortices on neuro patients, such as stroke, head injury and coma victims. I have observed that if Cortices is done on patients as soon as possible, they recover more quickly and require less rehabilitation. I have seen severe stroke patients regain function; and in many cases I am convinced that, without Cortices, they would have been going to a nursing home instead of back home to their families.

Another form of severe shock can be diagnosed as a coma. You can have coma from injury to the brain, and that is a different state of affairs in which the brain has physically been damaged. However, many forms of coma occur when the body has gone into a severe shock and not been able to come out of it. The injuries may have repaired internally, but the person is still lying in a hospital bed in a severe state of shock, which we call a coma. Again, clinically, we have had many cases in which hospitalized persons in comas have had their Cortices tapped out and come out of the coma – often within minutes or hours. Many have been in their coma for months or years. This is where BodyTalk can be a vital instrument to be used in hospital settings.

The other benefit of Cortices that I have seen over the years is for people who are in a chronic mild state of shock. Because of the daily stresses discussed earlier, these people have a blankness in the eyes, and, while the responses are there, they are not clear or sharp. These people can function at their basic job and even drive a car, but they are in this constant state of semi-shock, which is a sort of coping mechanism the body uses in order to dull the trauma of being in a stressed state.

Access after a Fall on Slippery Rocks
Suryo Gardner, CBI - Seattle, Washington, USA

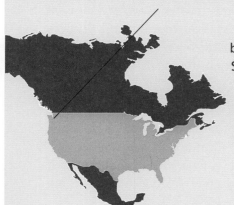

My friend, Sonja, fell in a ravine, into a pile of boulders, as we were out hiking on slippery rocks. She was bleeding and in shock, and it appeared that she had hit her head. I did Cortices and she immediately came out of shock. Within five minutes, she was able to stand and walk out of the ravine with me. She says I saved her life.

Cortices Technique for Car Sickness

Ben Manalo, CBI - Chicago, Illinois, USA

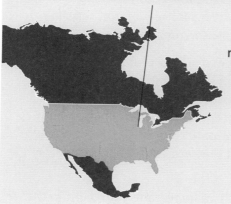

My niece was feeling car sick during a short ride to a baseball game. I turned around to ask if she wanted BodyTalk, but her mom already had started doing Cortices on her. When she finished tapping, the car sickness was gone.

The amygdalae (plural) are a pair of almond-shaped neural nuclei deep within the brain, which analyze neural stimuli based on its catalog of previous experiences, and can provide a shortcut to the fight-flight sympathetic nervous system switch, when a potential emergency is recognized.

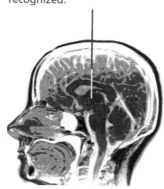

With BodyTalk, we are addressing these two fronts simultaneously: While the Cortices treatment helps repair the functioning of the **amygdala** system and its relationship to the thalamus, the hypothalamus, hippocampus, prefrontal cortex, etc. (which improves the body's ability to deal with stress), it can also bring someone out of shock so their brain can function far better.

When you bring someone out of a mild state of shock, it means they are going to repair their own body better. For example, when someone is in a state of mild shock, the brain is not going to be very observant. We are not just talking about being switched off to the world around you; we have to remember that, to the brain, the body is the world around it. We find that people very often will live with chronic viruses, infections, parasites or allergies because the body is in shock. Thus their immune systems are not observant enough to pick up the existence of those microbes in the body and therefore are not attacking them and killing them off. As a result, a person can live with fatigue, pain, headaches or what is sometimes diagnosed as Chronic Fatigue Syndrome or fibromyalgia because their defense systems are being compromised due to mild shock.

That is why we have found that just doing the Cortices technique alone can often precipitate a major repairing of the body, as the body starts spontaneously looking for microbes and killing them off. We also see injuries repair faster as the brain starts to function more clearly.

We have found this extremely important in children who have extremely poor attention spans. One of the problems is that they are living in a state of shock because of the stress they are under. This stress can come from their environment, their school facilities, family situations or even from the additives and toxins in the food they are eating or the medications they are taking.

This is why Cortices is such an important ingredient in the body's ability to start healing itself. We find that by tapping out the Cortices on a weekly or bi-weekly basis, we are gradually improving the body's resilience to handle stress and reducing its tendency to go into shock. We eventually can teach the body not to go into shock, except in cases in which it needs to due to extreme stress.

This concept is preventative medicine. By using BodyTalk Access on a regular basis, you will be improving the functioning of the brain and eventually the functioning of the body's built-in health maintenance systems, so that the person is less likely to get sick in the first place.

To help you understand the power of BodyTalk Access, I encourage you to learn the simple Cortices technique that follows, applying it on your friends and family and having them apply it on you. I guarantee you will notice the positive changes that occur.

If you are a practitioner and apply the Cortices technique before starting an acupuncture treatment, a massage, chiropractic or even drug therapy, you will find that, by balancing the hemispheres of the brain to work better, reducing the stress level and bringing the person out of a mild state of shock, the patient will respond far better to the therapy and heal much quicker.

Fast Aid to the Rescue in Austria

Sharon Gelber, Access Trainer - Sydney, Australia

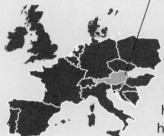

While traveling in Vienna, Austria, I happened to be passing by the Vienna Marathon, in which about 60,000 international runners annually compete. A female runner collapsed unconscious in the street right in front of me. I was immediately at her side applying Access techniques to stabilize her. These included continuously activating her brain (cortices), hydration and switching.

The ambulance and medics took some time to arrive and apply oxygen. Meanwhile the woman had slowly regained consciousness and then was taken to hospital.

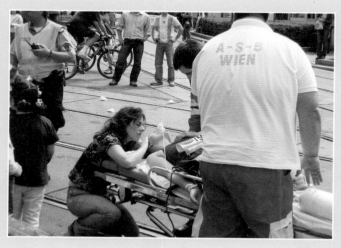

I would love to see a day when Cortices is a standard practice to start any form of therapy treatment. Even, for example, in counseling, where the person could be in a state of shock or stress overload and not hearing or correctly interpreting what is being said to them. If the two brain hemispheres are not going to be talking very effectively, the practitioner is not going to make a profound impact due to disjointed thinking and possible misinterpretation of what is being said. As a result, it could require many more sessions to get the same results.

Another use of this technique is to help with sports or academic performance. We have found that if you tap out the Cortices in a child who is about to undergo an exam or play a sport, they will perform far better because they have addressed the stress overload that often comes with a challenge. If we have children tapping out their Cortices just before they start a school day, before they take a test, before they are about to participate in a sport or perform in a play, it is going to make a very big difference. We have seen this already in trial studies we have done in various schools, where tapping out the Cortices at the beginning of the day has vastly improved the level of interaction between the students and the teacher, the behavior of the students, the children's ability to learn and a subsequent improvement in the grades of the class.

The Cortices technique being taught to children at the Sunshine School in Bali.

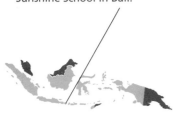

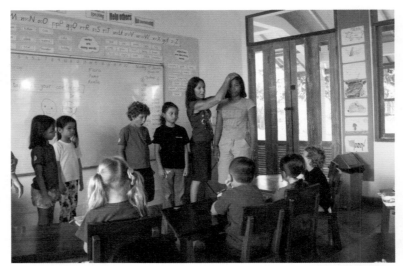

Oregon Access Experiment

Sandra Wenrich, Access Trainer - Portland, Oregon, USA

We ran an eight-week experiment in an elementary school in Oregon, in which both students and teachers received Access sessions twice a week. Here are a few remarks from the participants:

From the Children:

"BodyTalk really helps a lot of things, like math, recess, art. It helps my mind work out things. BodyTalk is an all around helper." 5th grade girl

"For eight weeks we had BodyTalk. It helped me not to get sick and to take away stress. It helps me to be more relaxed, joyful and kind." 6th grade boy

From the Parents:

"(My daughter)… likes your program. She has been happier and has adjusted more easily to the many life changes taking place."

"(My daughter)… seems to be doing better in spelling. Also when she had a cold, she was not sick for as long as in the past."

From a Teacher:

Regarding her own experience: "I am always so much more relaxed and grounded after a session. The reciprocals especially helped the balance within my body and helped me hold my chiropractic adjustments longer, too."

Regarding the children: "Most really enjoyed the sessions and those especially in need of greater balance/stability/calmness in their lives seemed to benefit the most. Although it seemed pretty chaotic and loud in the classroom during the sessions, the rest of the day tended to go more smoothly. Students were generally more cooperative with each other (and me) and in better control of themselves; more flexible too."

Now I am going to teach you how to tap out the Cortices. I encourage you to experiment with it to see its effectiveness for yourself.

Tapping strategic parts of the body is a fundamental principle in a number of healthcare modalities, some dating back to ancient times.

All BodyTalk techniques – including BodyTalk Access – rely on a tapping process to bring them into effect. The light tapping is used to facilitate the communication required and to store the memory of the changes that are being made. The tapping process involves spreading the fingers to reach over both hemispheres of the brain and gently tapping on the head. This alternates with the fingers lightly tapping over the center of the chest on the sternum to activate the energetic heart complex.

How to Tap

Tapping of the brain is accomplished by spreading the fingers and thumb so that both hemispheres are contacted across the midline of the skull. Tapping of the heart is done over the center of the chest on the sternum or breastbone with the focus on the heart underneath. All tapping is done lightly at a comfortable speed. Since this is an energetic movement, the tapping will still work even if the head or chest is not physically contacted at all. This is a consideration in areas of the world where it is culturally inappropriate to touch someone or even illegal to touch another person for therapeutic purposes.

The tapping is alternated between the brain and heart while the contact points are indicated energetically or physically held. It is not necessary to synchronize the tapping with the breathing.

Note that it is possible to access the heart energy not only by tapping on the sternum, but, if it is more convenient, by tapping on the back in between the shoulder blades. The heart's energy pattern is accessible from all sides!

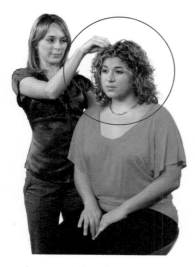 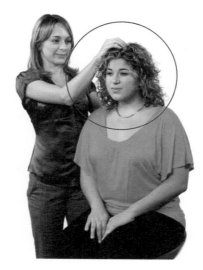

Incorrect Tapping: *Make sure both left and right hemispheres of the brain are contacted.*

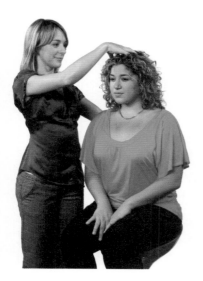 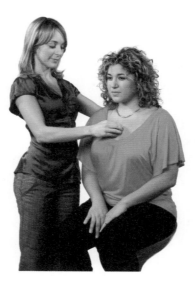 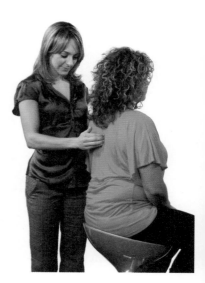

Correct Tapping: *Fingers spanning across both hemispheres of the brain*

Tapping the sternum

Tapping the back

The Cortices Technique: With A Partner

(A) Place one hand on the person's head at the base of the skull where it meets the neck. (Note: It is important to keep the fingers and thumb together throughout this technique to avoid missing any areas of the brain.) While holding that position, tap the head and then the sternum (or back) lightly, alternating for two full breath cycles.

Your focus while tapping out the Cortices is on connecting all points of the right hemisphere of the brain to the left hemisphere and highlighting and eliminating all the "cold spots" of diminished blood supply or cellular activity that are present.

(B) Now move your hand up onto the head to the position next to the one you just used. (You are going to systematically cover the whole head, one hand-width at a time.) In the new position, tap out the head and sternum, alternating for two full breaths.

(C) This procedure is repeated until you have covered the whole midline of the head from the base of the skull to just above the eyebrows. This could mean three hand-widths for a large hand to cover a small head or five hand-widths for a small hand to cover a larger head. The main objective is to make sure that the entire brain is covered. The hand positions may overlap to ensure that no areas are left untouched.

(D) Now cover the sides of the head to balance the temporal lobes. Preferably, have the person cover both sides of his or her head with their own hands. Or you can cover both sides of their head with your hands. Now tap out while the person takes two full breaths. (If you are doing it the second way, let go with one of your hands to tap the head and sternum [or back].)

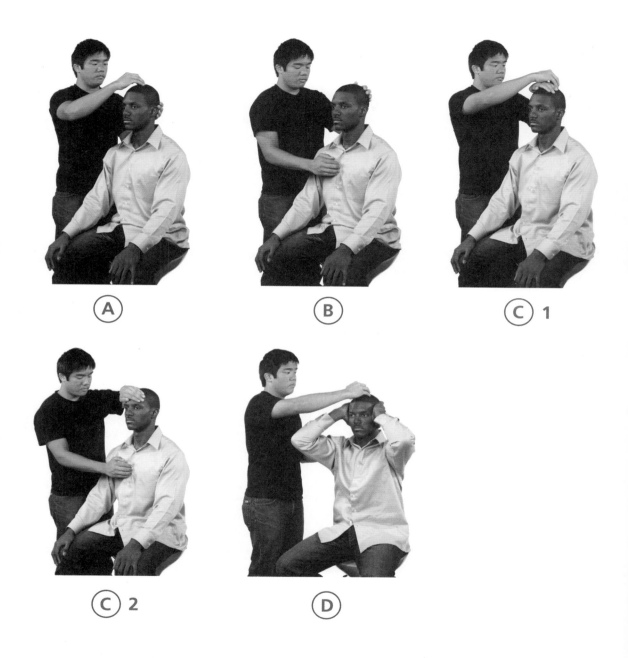

A

B

C 1

C 2

D

The Cortices Technique: Self-Application

(A) Place one hand, with fingers together, at the base of your skull, so that it straddles both sides of your head and covers the top of the neck and the bottom of the skull. While holding this position, tap the head and then the sternum with your other hand, alternating for two full breath cycles.

Your focus while tapping out the Cortices is on connecting all points of the right hemisphere of the brain to the left hemisphere and highlighting and eliminating all the "cold spots" of diminished blood supply or cellular activity that are present.

(B) Now move your hand up onto your head just above the position you just held. (You are going to systematically cover the whole head one hand-width at a time.) In the new position, tap out your head and sternum alternating for two full breaths.

(C) Repeat this procedure until you have covered the whole midline of the head from the base of your skull to just above your eyebrows, making sure that the entire brain is covered. Your hand positions may overlap to ensure that no areas are left untouched.

(D) Now cover the sides of your head to balance the temporal lobes of your brain. After holding both sides of your head for a few seconds, let go with one hand; and while still holding one side of your head, use your other hand to tap on your head and then on your sternum. After each head and sternum tapping, place your tapping hand back onto the side of your head for a few seconds. Continue this process for at least two full breath cycles.

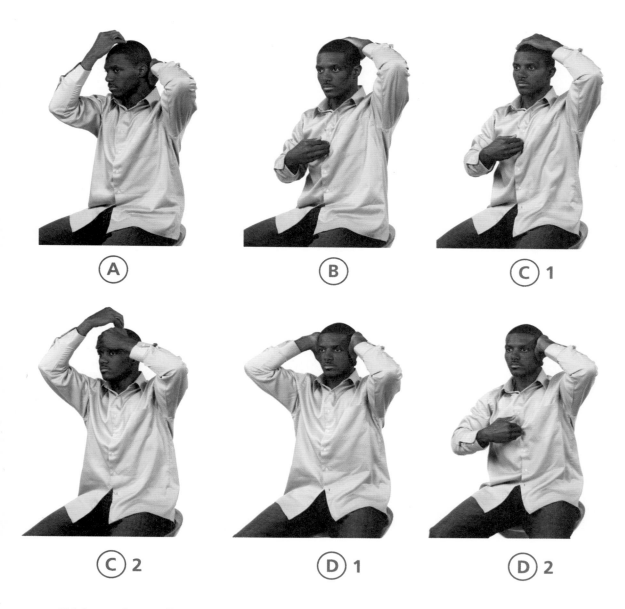

With regular application of this Cortices technique, you will find that your head may feel less "foggy," your mental focus may sharpen, or you may just feel more balanced and clear. Try it out. It can do no harm, and it has the potential to do so much good.

Switching

The Switching and Cortices techniques go closely hand in hand, because they can address many of the same symptoms of brain imbalance, shock and malfunction. Despite this relationship, however, switching is quite specific in its nature.

The prerequisite for the switching phenomenon is, in fact, a person being under stress. In other words, their cortices are not working and not communicating well. Switching is a natural mechanism to stop overload that, in a healthy person, works only when it is really necessary.

As an example, if you overtax yourself by working on a computer for hours without rest, nutrition, etc., you will get to a point at which you suddenly will go into a switched state, signaling that the functioning of the left and right hemispheres and the way they work in harmony with one another is severely compromised.

In this switched state, yes, you are in a state of shock, but you also are in a state in which you basically shut down. You find you cannot think clearly at all and cannot continue with your computer work because you are making mistakes galore, your typing has become erratic and you even are starting to feel ill. What your body is saying to you is that you have overdone it, your glucose levels are too low and you are extremely fatigued. Thus it has put you in a switched state so you will stop, have something to eat, have a rest and recharge. What switching does is keep you from becoming extremely ill by overtaxing the body.

"It felt like an elephant had jumped out of a tree onto my shoulders and was making me carry it the rest of the way in." - Dick Beardsley, speaking of hitting "the wall" after completing a marathon.

We can see the same concept in long-distance runners. When marathon runners **"hit the wall,"** they actually are switching. The runners' bodies are saying that they are overtaxed, the blood glucose levels are too low, their bodies have done too much work. Therefore, they go into a rather dazed state in which they feel that they cannot run any further, they lose concentration, etc. What marathon runners are trained to do, however, is go through that wall and come out the other side by going onto emergency reserves in the body.

Studies on Australian marathon runners at the Australian Institute of Sport have shown that from the time they switch and go through the "wall" onward, they are actually destroying their bodies. As a result, we often see that long-distance runners who "hit the wall" are people who get old very quickly. They often have many health problems later on in life because of the damage they have done. (Interestingly, this is not true, however, for persons with certain metabolisms, such as some Kenyan and Ethiopian runners, for example, who can run an entire marathon without "hitting the wall" and entering into a switched state.)

Competitive athletics aside, there are many aspects of life in which switching occurs, particularly under stress. A classic example of a switching situation is when someone asks you to raise your right hand and you put up your left. Or, when driving, you are directed to turn left and you turn right. Those are typical switching symptoms: getting everything back to front, doing the opposite of what you are supposed to be doing. In the mental processes, often you are saying "yes" when you mean "no." You often are making decisions that are the opposite of what they should be because there is confusion as to what is right and wrong.

Switching is your classic self-destruct mode.

When you are in a switched state, you cannot think clearly and there is a natural tendency to do the opposite of what is good for you. Thus, for instance, a person who is on a diet can reach a certain point of stress and switch, embarking on an eating binge. Or a person who is upset can be stressed to the point of seeking relief through drugs or alcohol.

Switching can be induced by a variety of factors, both personally unique and seemingly mundane.

Interestingly, one of the more tragic incidences we see involves strobe lighting. For example, it has been shown that when a fluorescent light in an office malfunctions and begins to flicker, it will cause anyone sitting under that light to go into a switched mode. This can cost a company a fortune, as employees in a switched mode make mistake after mistake after mistake, and their output is diminished. This situation continues until the light is repaired or replaced, as employees operating in a switched state continue to make incorrect decisions. Further, if something is not done quickly, affected employees go into the cortices coping mode of shutting down into a state of mild shock.

The same thing can happen in a classroom, profoundly affecting the children in the vicinity of the flickering lights.

Another example is found in night clubs and dance venues with strobe lighting. In those environments, healthy, well-balanced people under a bit of stress and already in a state of shock can immediately go into switched mode. In this switched mode, they may start to do the exact opposite of what they normally would mean to do. They will, for instance, go into a self-destruct mode of overdrinking, getting involved with drugs or just doing stupid things. This is a very serious situation, and we see this self-destruct mode occurring very clearly in these types of situations.

However it is induced, switching has a profound impact on its sufferers.

Because of their stress levels, many people switch too easily, going in and out of switch mode almost every day and even several times a day and hence making mistakes and impractical decisions, not thinking clearly and malfunctioning.

For example, one symptom of switching is dyslexia. You will find that when you have dyslexic children and "unswitch" them, they may no longer be dyslexic. However, they can quickly revert to the dyslexia because they switch too easily when under stress, such as when they have to read. In such a case, a practitioner will have to do the Switching and the Cortices techniques in combination over a period of time to gradually strengthen the brain and heighten its stress threshold, so the body will not switch as easily and will be far more functional on a day-to-day basis.

It is critical to note that in BodyTalk Access, the treatment is not designed to permanently "unswitch" anyone. It can "unswitch" someone who is in switched mode at the time of treatment, of course, and, if done over a period of time on a regular basis, it can heighten the person's threshold for switching. That said, we do not want to eliminate the body's ability to switch because it is a natural mechanism that can save a person's life during periods of extreme stress.

In discussing switching, I have been talking a lot about children because it can be so obvious in them. For instance, parents have learned to cope with a child's dyslexia by not forcing him or her to read or do other things that create switching. The average person, however, lives in this chronic state of coping by going into mild shock, coming in and out of switching almost all the time and compromising the immune system.

You can imagine the value of these two techniques – Switching and Cortices – and their vital importance to quality of life and just being able to exist in this world in a much more lucid way with far better cognition of what is going on and the ability to think clearly, respond effectively and work and play in a constructive way.

Hydration

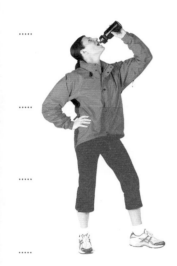

Hydration has become quite a catchword these days, as you see people walking around with their water bottles, trying to keep their fluids up. Unfortunately, however, this is not necessarily solving any problems.

Although there have been some great books on the subject of hydration, one I recommend is *Your Body's Many Cries for Water* by Fereydoon Batmanghelidj, M.D. This book emphasizes that we have to realize that our bodies are up to 80 percent water, and water is absolutely critical for the body's functioning.

NOTHING OCCURS WITHOUT WATER

Two-thirds of the human body is made up of water, H_2O, with cells consisting of 65-90% water by weight. This body water is distributed in different compartments in the body. Lean muscle tissue contains about 75% water. Blood contains 83% water, body fat contains 25% water and bone has 22% water.

The nervous system requires water for the transportation of electrons and proper communication and functioning. The brain is 80 percent water. Every nerve pathway has a micro-tubule of water that, if not there, will negatively affect the functioning of the nervous system.

Water is also the main ingredient for cells to generate energy; in fact, water is part and parcel in energy production in the body. In addition, water is the main transporter of nutrition, vitamins, etc., through cell membranes. You could have plenty of good nutrition, but, without water, your ability to take that nutrition into your cells would be compromised.

This means you could eat very well but actually be mal-nourished.

The existence and actions of water molecules also control the metabolism for emotions and the functioning of the muscles and the connective tissue, which is so critical in the storage of memory for movement.

In BodyTalk, we have discovered that people can drink a lot of water but still be dehydrated. The concept is that we can detect in these people all the signs of dehydration – poor energy, poor metabolism, poor nutrition, poor functioning of the nervous system, a highly stressed and volatile nervous system, dry skin and so on – which means that, though they may be drinking plenty of water, the water is not getting to the places where it is needed. Rather, the water is staying between the cells. In fact, such persons also could have edema (swelling caused by too much water in the tissues), as a result of the water taken in but not utilized properly by the body. In other words, the mechanism that enables the water to be utilized by the nervous system or for it to be able to transport nutrition or other elements across the cell membranes has been compromised.

The BodyTalk technique for Hydration is designed to address that problem: to get the water to be utilized properly by the cells; to increase the transportation of water molecules across the cell membranes; to be able to hold the water molecules with the correct electrical charge around all the cells, in the connective tissue and along the neurological pathways.

IT IS NOT ABOUT THE QUANTITY OF WATER; IT IS ABOUT THE QUALITY OF THE USE OF THE WATER WE HAVE IN THE BODY.

We have found that once we have done the Hydration techniques on people, they immediately start responding by showing signs of better nutrition, better functioning of the nervous system, far less stress in the system and so on. Often, the demand or need for water is diminished, and they find they do not have to drink as much and, in fact, they are not as thirsty.

The unfortunate situation is that so many people are thirsty all the time because their bodies are screaming for water, but the water they take in is not getting to the cells. Once we do the Hydration technique, often their excessive thirst stops, their metabolism improves, the excess water between the cells diminishes, they lose weight and so on.

The problem of poor hydration has been amplified in modern Western societies. Here we see a rapidly growing trend for children to drink less water. Instead, they drink caffeinated soft drinks that act as diuretics and cause even greater dehydration. Hence, they have poor absorption of foods and a tendency to have malfunctions of the nervous system due to the diminished nerve conduction. This contributes to hyperactivity, learning disorders and compromised immune systems.

Hydration is a critical factor for any health situation. Your body simply cannot respond and heal properly unless the water molecules in it are being effectively utilized. This technique in BodyTalk Access is designed to insure that effective utilization.

Body Chemistry

Body Chemistry is one of the original techniques in BodyTalk and, along with Cortices, would be considered the most commonly used and most valuable technique. Essentially, the Body Chemistry technique is designed to get the immune system to respond appropriately to things that are going wrong within the body. It was a prototype version of the Body Chemistry technique that helped my body overcome the Epstein-Barr virus years ago.

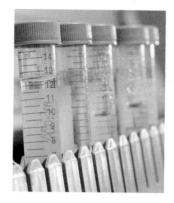

"U.S. researchers have identified all 1,116 unique proteins found in human saliva glands, a discovery they said on Tuesday could usher in a wave of convenient, spit-based diagnostic tests that could be done without the need for a single drop of blood.

As many as 20 percent of the proteins that are found in saliva are also found in blood, said Fred Hagen, a researcher at the University of Rochester Medical Center in New York who worked on the study".
- Julie Steenhuysen of *Scientific American*

Our bodies are full of microbes. Many of them, of course, are good bacteria doing a good job. Others, however, are harmful bacteria, viruses or parasites that sometime announce their presence in what we call an infection. In addition, the body has a tendency to hold on to harmful microbes for extended periods of time – creating a chronic situation that is irritating to the immune system and to the body and can compromise the body's healthy functioning.

Today, throughout the world, there are many people who have chronic low-grade infections, viruses and parasites present in their bodies, that are weakening their immune systems and causing a great a deal of malfunctioning and health problems.

The Body Chemistry technique is designed to systematically help the body gradually fight all these detrimental microbes and eliminate them from the system. We do this by taking a sample of the patient's **saliva** and putting it on the navel. This allows the immune system, at an energic level, to pick up many problems that it would not see at the straight physiological level because they are so well hidden.

Modern science has shown that the saliva contains the energic blueprint of virtually everything that is happening in the body and particularly the blueprints of all the disease processes that are going on. At this energic level, the body actually can measure these detrimental changes and then bring about the appropriate physiological generation of antibodies or antigens that will then eliminate the particular problems.

This Body Chemistry technique that we teach in Access is a simplified version that has to be done fairly regularly so the body can systematically work through its various problems. With this version, we cannot specifically target a particular microbe or a particular parasite, as we can in the advanced levels of BodyTalk. However, we have found that whenever there is an acute situation, such as someone's coming down with the flu or getting a bit of food poisoning from harmful bacteria, then when we use this technique the immune system will give that acute condition a priority.

So the wonderful thing about this technique is that, in any community or family, when anyone becomes sick through some form of invasive process of microbes, we can get the immune system to effectively fight it off very quickly – much quicker than it normally would. For instance, if a young child with a virus such as the flu is treated using BodyTalk Access, the illness often will be gone within a day or so vs. a week or two. So, this obviously is a powerful technique.

Another major benefit of the Body Chemistry technique is that it works on food intolerances or food allergies, where a person is reacting to a type or class of food. By using the Body Chemistry technique in combination with the rest of the Access techniques, we can quickly train the body's immune system to overcome this reaction and correct the intolerance. This is extremely important to many people who react very strongly to different types of food.

This also goes for environmental allergies, such as when people overreact to substances such as pollen, with symptoms that are more pronounced in degree and duration. In such cases, we have found that the Body Chemistry technique will help the immune system to stabilize this process and dramatically reduce or even eradicate the allergy.

Fast Aid for Recurrent Acid Reflux

Brett Selby - Matlock, Derbyshire, UK

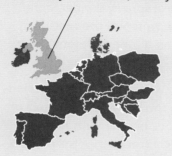

Enjoying life on Curbar Edge in the UK.

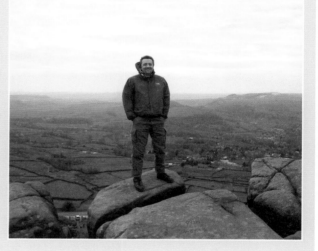

I had a bad acute episode of this longstanding and painful problem and was considering different self-treatment options when I remembered Fast Aid. I linked the Cortices to the esophagus, and there was an 80-percent immediate improvement. I feel so relieved to know there is something I can do to help myself on the spot!

By creating a system to treat allergies, food intolerances and parasites, harmful viruses and bacteria in a very simple and safe way, without the use of antibiotics and other drugs, we have established a very efficient form of healthcare that will tackle most of the simple cases. I should stress that, in cases of severe infection – whether it be bacterial infection or very severe parasitical infection, drugs sometimes are also necessary. The beauty of BodyTalk Access is that we will know very quickly if additional healthcare treatment is needed because if Access is enough, we will see definite improvement in 24 hours. Thus, if the person is actually worse in 24 hours, then we know the immune system is not strong enough to tackle this on its own, and it would be best to use the appropriate drug or other healthcare therapy.

Another very important aspect of Body Chemistry is seen in the buildup of toxins in the system. In this day and age, we have become very aware of all the different types of pollutants, such as exhaust fumes, chemical sprays, dander, mold, mercury from dental fillings; the detrimental products in cigarette smoke; lead poisoning, and all the different chemicals that are affecting our lives.

The Body Chemistry technique, when done over a period of time, is very effective in getting the body to clear itself of these toxins. We have seen numerous people with mercury or lead poisoning or suffering effects from other toxins who, after the use of BodyTalk for a short period of time, have had those detrimental toxins eliminated from their systems – with all the symptoms associated with them gone, as well.

So, all in all, Body Chemistry is one of the most powerful techniques and powerful tools that anyone can have, and anyone who learns it will be successful in enhancing the quality of life of their family or community.

Reciprocals

The Reciprocals represent the most involved technique to learn in the BodyTalk Access program. That is because mastery of Reciprocals involves memorizing quite a few places on the body that we have to touch in pairs in order to bring about changes. Essentially, the Reciprocals involve the musculoskeletal functioning of the body.

Among the fascinating work that is coming out nowadays is the discovery that the body works quite differently than we originally thought.

We have always tended to think that the skeleton holds the body together, the muscles move the skeleton, we have discs and joints in the spine for weight bearing and so on. And yet the latest discoveries have shown that the body actually works in the same way as the engineering concept of tensegrity.

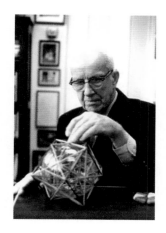

R. Buckminster Fuller (July 12, 1895 – July 1, 1983) was an American architect, author, designer, futurist, inventor, poet and visionary. He wrote more than thirty books, coining and popularizing terms such as Spaceship Earth, ephemeralization, and synergetics.

Tensegrity is a term employed by one of the most famous engineering architects, **Buckminster Fuller,** who used this principle in the development of his geodesic domes and many other structures, whereby having pulleys and wires and all the right weights, you create self-supporting systems that do not apply excessive pressure in any one particular spot.

What researchers now have discovered is that the human musculo-skeletal system works as a transegrity matrix, as well, because all the ligaments, muscles and fascia of the body, as well as the angles in which they are organized (i.e. in spiral forms and with various attachments), work in a way that is very different than we ever thought.

In fact, the body stands because of this dynamic transegrity matrix and balance of the muscular patterns of the body to the point that if the body is very healthy, there is very minimal pressure on areas such as the intevertebral discs of the spine and the menisci of the knees. What researchers actually have shown is that the spine as we walk and move is being held together in a dynamic that does not involve heavy pressure on the discs, and therefore would not wear out a disc in a healthy system. In a healthy body, joints should be under tension rather than compression.

It is only when the transegrity of the body is compromised – for instance, because of malfunctioning of the muscles or thickening of the fascia through scar tissue – that the transegrity complex collapses and we start weight bearing and putting pressure on the discs and other joints as we walk. And that, of course, would cause the discs to wear down and wear out. This is a major cause of pain and degenerative problems in the back, hips, knees and ankles.

The latest discoveries purport that, rather than cutting the knee cartilage and doing reconstruction, re-establishment of the transegrity balance of the body would automatically take the pressure off the discs involved and create a negative pressure. In fact, that would then encourage the disc to regenerate itself. It now has been shown that if you actually take the pressure off the disc and create a negative force or vacuum in the knee, the cartilage in the knee actually will grow back, eliminating the need for surgery or joint replacement.

We find also that the structure of the body and how well this transegrity matrix works is very much a part of the general healthy functioning of the whole body. That is because the movement of the muscles and fascia of the body stimulates the functions of the organs and, in fact, this transegrity matrix goes right into the very depths of the body at a cellular level. Within the cells of the body, there is a connective tissue transegrity matrix that is quite complex and is the major factor in biochemical reactions and physiological functioning of the body.

In BodyTalk, we take great note of this and, in our advanced work, we tend to focus on the transegrity balance of connective tissue within cells, fascia and muscles.

The Reciprocals are the beginning of this. They are the overview, where we look at the gross structure of the body and the dynamic balance between its various parts, for example, the relationship between the opposing parts of the body from the distance of the navel, such as the left shoulder to the right hip. We have found that if people have right-hip problems, they also have/will have imbalances and problems in the left shoulder and vice versa. This is true with the right elbow and left knee, and so on.

These combinations of points that usually are on opposite sides and opposite ends of the body are what we call reciprocal points. We have found that by balancing these points, by touching the Reciprocals and doing our process of tapping on the head and tapping on the chest, we can help to re-establish the transegrity balance and dynamics of the posture, which, in turn, improves the posture and functioning of the body. As the body starts functioning with more efficiency and with improved balance, the person will be walking better and sitting better, and this means all the connective tissue of the body is going to operate better, the circulation will be better, and the flow of the electrons and protons in the connective tissue, the flow of nerve impulses, the circulation, the lymph drainage and all the different functions of the entire body are going to improve.

So while balancing of the Reciprocals is very simple, its first immediate effect is a major change in the health of the body from a mechanical point of view. By first improving the posture of the spine, we eliminate much of the pain that people experience from poor body posture and promote repair of the spine.

But, more importantly, by balancing the Reciprocals, we also are improving the general function of every aspect of the body right down to the chemical equations that occur inside its cells. Therefore, this transegrity principle is extremely important for us.

At the Access level, we tend to use a much simpler approach that is global, while, in advanced BodyTalk, we go into it much more deeply at a micro level.

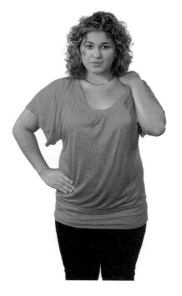

The shoulder and the opposite hip are just one of several important pairs of Reciprocal points in the body.

Fast Aid

There is one other technique taught in the BodyTalk Access course that we call Fast Aid. This protocol can be very effective in dealing with minor emergencies or in stabilizing someone while waiting for emergency aid to arrive in the case of a more serious emergency. Of course, we always advise that anyone encountering a serious emergency situation follow all appropriate first aid guidelines.

But the Fast Aid protocol, which consists of tapping out the Cortices, then once again tapping out the Cortices while linking to the injured area, and then linking the injured area to its Reciprocal point, very often can stimulate the body to rapidly initiate its self-healing capabilities. When in doubt, simply tapping out the Cortices, as frequently as deemed appropriate, can go a long way toward bringing the body into self-healing mode.

Fast Aid for Injured Hand
Patricia Gast, CBP - Littleton, Colorado, USA

A client had slammed her right hand in a car door and was holding ice on it when I walked in. Her hand was red and purple in color and had a "bubble" forming and growing in size on the back of it. She seemed to be scared, in pain and in slight shock. I performed the Fast Aid protocol for 20 minutes, after which the client reported having less pain and stiffness, due to a decrease in swelling and inflammation. In addition, the "bubble" disappeared, there was an increase in range of motion in her grip and the color of her hand returned to normal. Her overall color returned, as well, and the client was noticeably relaxed, with no sign of shock.

Fast Aid for Burn

Donna Kozoriz, CBP - Edmonton, Alberta, Canada

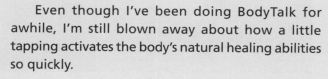

Even though I've been doing BodyTalk for awhile, I'm still blown away about how a little tapping activates the body's natural healing abilities so quickly.

For instance, we had a birthday party for our neighbour. I was stir-frying the chicken, and I put too much oil in the wok, then stirred it too quickly while I was yakking. As a result, I splashed enough oil on my toes to fill my sandal – boiling oil. I immediately started Fast Aid.

People were running around, starting cars to take me to the hospital, and I kept tapping. I raised my foot up, stuck it in the sink, ran water on it and tapped Cortices linked to my poor toes. The pain went away, and I kept tapping. The swelling stopped, and I kept tapping. I tapped for about five minutes.

A friend who has been skeptical about BodyTalk and was watching with "that" look, walked over and picked up my partially melted rubber sandal still full of oil. He then looked at my toes and said, "Holy #%$@ Donna; you're freaking me out!"

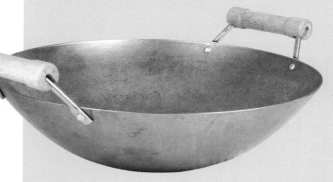

By the end of the day, my foot looked as though I had a sunburn – instead of the third-degree burns I would have had if I hadn't known Fast Aid. I'm so thankful.

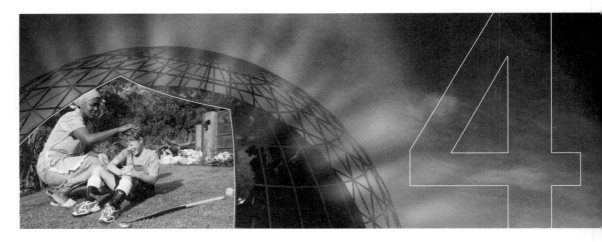

Chapter 4   **The World Health Crisis and Cost Factors**

It has become increasingly obvious that most of the world, from the developing countries to advanced Western nations such as Australia and the United States, are rapidly heading toward a healthcare crisis that, in turn, is also precipitating an economic crisis.

While the latter enjoy the benefits of all the new technology and sophisticated equipment that has been a boon to helping save lives, they also are bearing the dramatically increased costs of delivery of modern healthcare services.

This trend is not leveling out; in fact, it seems to be increasing almost out of control. This presents one of the major problems existing in countries such as the United States and one that is going to get worse, not better, unless something positive is done about it.

Already in the United States, a record 45 million people did not have healthcare insurance in 2006, generally due to lack of opportunity or ability to pay, and thus are in a serious situation if they get sick or hurt. With serious illnesses and injuries, some would likely have to declare bankruptcy or sell their homes to pay the medical bills. This, of course, is unacceptable.

In Third World countries, the situation is worse. In these nations, many millions of people are dying purely because there is no access to any form of significant healthcare that could save their lives.

There is also a trend in densely populated and poorer nations such as India to not want to take on the typical U.S. medical model, because they very well know that neither their poverty-stricken citizens nor their government can afford an advanced medical system with all the testing, laboratories and equipment, surgeries and drugs it encompasses.

Wherever our locations on the globe, therefore, it has become increasingly obvious that we have to go back to some form of an entry-level healthcare system that covers the simpler things in a very cost-effective manner.

Providing Access sessions for the Orang Asli Tribe in the jungles of Malaysia

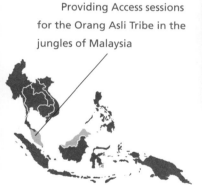

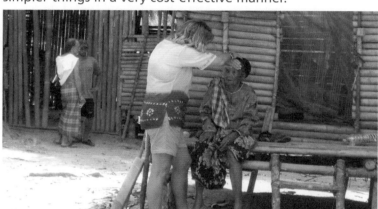

This is where, I feel, BodyTalk Access comes in.

My belief is based on the fact that a person who is treated on a regular basis to keep his or her system functioning well is going to have far fewer health problems. This concept of preventative medicine is talked about a lot. Unfortunately, however, many of the things we actually do about it have limited application, and some people do not have the luxury of good diets, proper exercise and so on. Whether they are uninformed or impoverished or just too busy or tired, people are not doing what they should to maintain good health.

The BodyTalk Access system is designed to help remedy that situation.

If Access is used within families and communities on a regular basis, it is going to continually upgrade people's general health by improving their brain function and strengthening their immune systems. As a result, they will have higher resistance to the various microbes that may come and go seasonally and an enhanced ability to maintain good health. And even when they do get sick, they should need far less, and less costly, medical attention.

An effective preventative maintenance system would, in fact, save countries billions of dollars a year just by reducing the demand for all the sophisticated healthcare systems.

I feel very strongly that if nations, communities and families were to utilize the BodyTalk Access system as part of their daily routines, they could dramatically improve their quality of life and reduce the need for costly healthcare services, saving everyone a great deal of money, while helping them live their lives more fully.

Obviously we will still need medicine as we know it today for the more serious cases, but at least under this approach of promoting health maintenance and treating simple disorders with simple techniques such as BodyTalk Access, we are freeing the doctors to do what they do best. And that is emergency medical care and treatment of serious conditions that require the sophistication of modern, mainstream medicine.

At this stage, I believe we need to convert from purely symptomatic treatment and dealing with health problems to the concept of well-being, quality of life and health maintenance.

Once we have done that, we will see a dramatic turn-around in the march toward a global healthcare crisis and a vast improvement in the way communities interact with one another. Their general well-being will ensure that they will be far less prone to the amygdala crisis of fear and anger and will have far healthier immune systems and brain function.

Access for Hornet Sting

Linda Kaczmar - Fort Frances, Ontario, Canada

We recently took our 4-year-old grand-daughter, Mikayla, fishing, and she got stung by a hornet. The week before, she had watched me do Fast Aid on her mother, and I had done a complete BodyTalk Access procedure on her dad. So she knew what it was all about and had seen how it had immediately taken her mommy's pain away.

She was crying and screaming with pain and holding on to her leg as I began Fast Aid. I sat her on my lap, and I tapped her back rather than her front, as it was more accessible that way. Her pain stopped almost immediately and she stopped screaming. I finished Fast Aid, and she was okay.

I didn't even think about how to go about doing it, I just did it immediately; it was like it was second nature to me. If I hadn't known BodyTalk Fast Aid, we would have had to come in from the lake right away, as we were dealing with a small child.

Thank God for BodyTalk Fast Aid and that I have taken the BodyTalk Access course. I have used it on myself all summer, too, for different things. It's absolutely amazing! I wish my siblings would be open to it. I thank God that my children and my husband are not closed-minded, and I am able to help them.

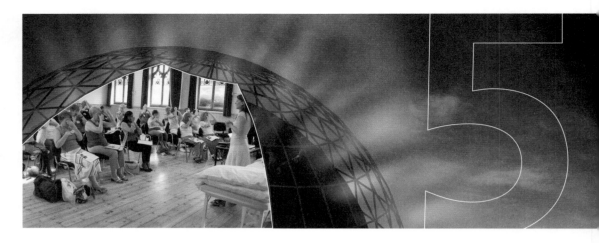

Chapter 5 Uses of BodyTalk Access

The role of BodyTalk Access throughout the world has many different facets, several of which I already have discussed. I now would like to provide a general summary and some of the ways in which we have seen BodyTalk Access being utilized by societies in everyday life.

First, however, I would point out that utilizing BodyTalk Access means using some of the basic techniques, such as Cortices, as an ongoing preventative maintenance treatment and using its additional other aspects in more specific circumstances, such as when an illness arises and a full Access treatment is required.

You may think this maintenance aspect is a fairly hard thing to achieve; but, quite frankly, once people get into a routine of getting their Cortices tapped out, it can become a habit just like cleaning their teeth every day as preventative maintenance for keeping their teeth and gums healthy. In the latter case, people recognize the connection between their actions and results and have adopted a routine that they know very well is going to save them a great deal of money in dental costs and help spare them the pain of serious tooth and gum problems.

With the right education, we similarly could have people using the concept of tapping out the Cortices as part of a daily routine to prevent illness in their own body and to maintain a healthier lifestyle, with this ritual making a very big difference in the lives of families and communities.

As far as the full Access protocol, which involves all the other aspects of treating hydration and balancing out the hemispheres and boosting the immune system, we see many uses for it, most of which will be summarized in this chapter

Family and Communities

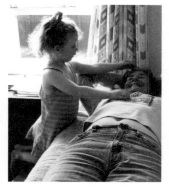

I already have talked about this quite a bit, but obviously the family and communities are very high on our agenda. That is because we would love to see someone in each family able to do the BodyTalk Access program to help maintain a healthy family unit and address 50 to 60 percent of simple health problems, thereby maximizing their quality of life. This would contribute greatly to the health of the communities and, of course, greatly diminish healthcare costs for them. Access also would reduce a tremendous amount of suffering because of its ability to prevent illnesses or to treat them at an early stage and get a very fast response. As noted, when average microbes such as a virus or an infection are treated with Access as soon as they occur, the sufferer often will be better within hours or the following day.

My 3-year old grand-daughter Janey just loves BodyTalk. When she was just 18 months, she was tapping the babies at her pre-school. Now when she comes to visit, she asks for a session, then gives me one. On this day I had another BodyTalker at my house, and she snapped this photo of Janey practicing BodyTalk on me. - Phillippa Peddie, New Zealand

Access will also have a significant effect on chronic pain such as arthritis. Regular Access sessions will greatly reduce the need for pain-killing drugs.

Hospitals and Rehabilitation

In the hospital setting, the scope of BodyTalk is unlimited. If we can have nurses trained in the BodyTalk program and utilizing BodyTalk Access on patients on a regular basis – particularly daily – we will see many things happen.

We will see the quality of life of patients improve as their suffering drastically diminishes. Plus, since the Access program is designed to speed up the entire healing process, we will see people recovering more quickly with far fewer side effects and complications.

For people who have terminal illnesses and are permanently in a hospital, the treatment of the Cortices and the balancing of the body and mind are going to improve their quality of life and even their quality of dying.

We have seen the effects of Access many times, while treating people who are suffering quite a lot, very stressed out, basically lying in the hospital waiting to die. After family members have used the basic BodyTalk Access program on these types of patients, a dramatic difference has been seen by both the family and the medical staff, as the patients ask for fewer painkillers, sleep better and seem far less stressed and far more comfortable, even happy.

Another aspect of this work is rehabilitation. After many types of surgery, such as hip replacements or knee repairs, rehabilitation can be slow, especially for middle-aged or older patients whose brains have been compromised and whose bodies and circuits are not operating as well as they could.

We have found that, when BodyTalk is used as part of the rehabilitation process, the results are greatly improved and the time needed to be devoted to rehab drastically reduced. In fact, we have seen that what normally could take weeks for rehabilitation often takes mere days when BodyTalk is included in the regimen. The beauty of BodyTalk is that it is easy to train nursing staff or even nursing aides to use these techniques. Training costs would be absolutely minimal, but the savings in having people respond better and complete rehab faster would be astronomical.

Nursing Homes

We see the same issue in nursing homes. Many people are in nursing homes for rehabilitation, but they often find that they never get well enough to go home. Our experience with BodyTalk is that when patients are treated in situations such as this, very often they are going to go home – joining their families or even going to their own residences to look after themselves.

So that is one big plus.

The other is that for people who are permanently in nursing homes due to serious illness or injury, the use of BodyTalk Access on them on a regular basis will improve their quality of life to a very large extent. Further, this will make the jobs of the doctors and other medical staff who are looking after these people far better and far more rewarding when they see their patients far less stressed, needing fewer pain killers and having a much happier personality dynamic.

Addiction Centers

BodyTalk can play a key role in helping people overcome many forms of addiction.

There are two aspects to this. One is the utilization of BodyTalk Access to reduce addicts' stress levels. This helps to clarify their thinking and to balance out the amygdala complex and the function of the nucleus accumbens, the pleasure center of the brain, which helps to keep their serotonin and dopamine levels in the right balance.

For people having a real battle with alcohol or drug withdrawal, simply training them to do the Cortices on themselves or each other on a routine basis will allow them to reap the benefits of the peace and clarity they receive, helping the whole process along.

Of course, patients with severe addictions also could be referred to an advanced BodyTalk practitioner, who would have a much larger range of practice and could use advanced BodyTalk techniques that are specific to helping to treat all the underlying complications of addictions, such as emotional aspects and history dynamics, as well as actual chemical reactions and physiological reactions to the drugs and drug withdrawal.

This is where the advanced levels of BodyTalk can play a huge role.

My own personal experience with this is watching and treating alcohol addiction. From a modern medicine point of view, it appears that the main aspect of alcohol addiction treatment is to get the people off the alcohol and send them to support groups and therapy designed to help them stay off. In other words, they live with their condition, but, under that circumstance, they are never allowed to have alcohol and they have a constant life struggle to overcome their addiction and maintain a clean life.

Under the BodyTalk System, we have found that if we treat the underlying factors – the key factors from fetal life though childhood and adult life, that is, the emotional factors – and then we treat the body chemistry and balance all the factors out, not only will the persons no longer be alcoholics but they do not even have to worry about drinking alcohol or not. In other words, I have treated many alcoholics who now can still have a glass of wine with their meal or have an occasional few drinks at a party, and they are not alcoholics. Drinking no longer causes them to be destructive to both themselves and those around them. This happens because I have actually treated the addiction and enabled them to live normal lives that include the occasional alcoholic drink.

It is very important to realize that we should not be branding people if they have that tendency. It is a treatable condition, and it just needs maintenance with the BodyTalk Access program and, in the initial stages, some advanced BodyTalk techniques to treat all the underlying causes so that the recovery is total from whatever the addiction is.

Paramedical

I mentioned a paramedical aspect earlier in the book, and I will just reiterate that we consider it extremely important that all paramedics be trained in at least BodyTalk Access. Using the Cortices technique can immediately bring people out of shock, while helping the body stabilize itself so it can control internal bleeding and regulate all the different body functions. This is an extremely important component of BodyTalk Access.

I also would point out what the paramedics I know have told me. When they go to crime or accident scenes and encounter people who have been severely injured or killed, this is highly stressful for them. Paramedics live in a very stressful state, so one of the major aspects of having them trained in BodyTalk Access is so, when they come back from a scene, they can tap each other out and help clear the stress out of their own minds and get rid of some of the shock they went into from the experience. I have seen so many cases of paramedics with post-traumatic stress disorder as a result of their work. By using BodyTalk Access on a regular basis, however, this can be prevented.

Access Reaches Taiwan

Karla Kadlec - Access Trainer, Calgary, Alberta, Canada

Last month I had the pleasure of teaching the first Access classes in Taiwan. The class was translated into Chinese for clarity and everyone enjoyed the hands-on approach to healing. There are now 20 Access Technicians in total and they are very keen to put their new knowledge to good use.

One week after our final class, my coordinator wrote this story to me about a newly graduated Access Technician: I heard secondhand about a story from Antonia. Walking on the street, she came upon a group waiting on an ambulance for an old man. Antonia did Cortices on him and when the ambulance came he sent the ambulance away and walked away. I saw Antonia today briefly and didn't hear the story other than her beaming about it and saying "I have no proof that what I did was the cause of him doing this, but the events happened in just this way."

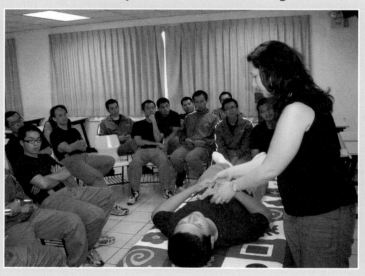

In addition to teaching the Access classes I was invited to many different organizations to give talks and demos on the BodyTalk System. The Taiwan Firefighter Training Center was one of these groups; they are very interested in making Access part of their standard training. The word "magic" was used to describe the quick changes the firefighters felt in their own bodies once Cortices were tapped out. They recognize the benefit this training would have for themselves as well as people in emergency situations. I look forward to working with this group again in the future.

Soldiers

In this day and age, we are seeing that the nature of the different wars going on around the world, particularly in Iraq, places a great deal of stress on the soldier. This is not to say that there has not been stress in previous wars, but it has become very evident that post-traumatic stress disorder is a very serious problem for returning soldiers. Quite frankly, they can accumulate many stresses while they are on duty, and when they come back we have a major problem in trying to reverse their effects.

I personally have treated many soldiers with post-traumatic stress disorder with a great deal of success. Unfortunately, once it is very severe and has been there for awhile, I tend to need the advanced BodyTalk techniques. However, so much of this could be neutralized if the soldiers, as part of their training, were taught the very basic techniques of BodyTalk Access. Then, in the field when they return from a maneuver, the soldiers could immediately tap each other out. This simple routine, which takes only a few minutes, could repair a great deal of damage from the stress and shock they have experienced. This would halt the accumulated stress in their systems, and I am absolutely certain it would have a dramatic effect on the soldiers' quality of life – and work. Even more importantly, it would enhance their ability to come back into society and function as totally normal individuals and not become people who, for the rest of their lives, develop personality and character disorders from post-traumatic stress.

The first-aid aspect of BodyTalk Access also can be extremely useful in combat zones, addressing simple things such back pain from lifting or spasms from sudden movements. The use of the Reciprocals in BodyTalk Access often can relieve such back pain within minutes and certainly rehabilitate the back and return it to good health within a day or two. And soldiers can do this on each other, rather than having to be taken to the medic, which often just does not happen. In many instances, they just take a lot of pain killers and learn to live with it. And, of course, the first aid capabilities of the Access techniques to bring wounded soldiers out of shock can save lives.

Pre- and Post-operation

As I mentioned earlier, we would love to see BodyTalk used much more in hospitals. However, not all operations are done in a hospital scenario; they often are done as outpatient services or in specialized clinics.

No matter the setting, though, we have found that if patients undergo the basic BodyTalk Access program before and after the operation, surgeons notice a significant difference in their recovery rates. They seem to recover far faster, have far fewer complications and come out of anesthesia with fewer side effects, such as nausea. This balancing also has the potential for shorter courses of pain medications and antibiotics as the healing process is stimulated. This is a very important component of Access that should be taken advantage of by all clinics, particularly when they are doing outpatient surgery.

Access to Speed Recovery from Surgery

Malcolm Thornton - Katikati, New Zealand

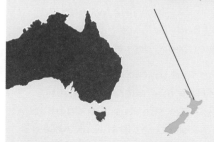

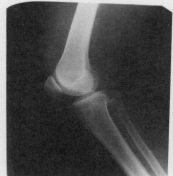

Many years ago, during a knee operation, the surgeon removed the wrong cartilage! I suffered pain ever since and in 2006 a total knee replacement was recommended (by a different surgeon).

My darling wife suggested I see a BodyTalker. Being the world's biggest skeptic, I reluctantly agreed to embark on this new (to me) form of therapy and subsequently had a BodyTalk session before being admitted to the hospital and another straight after the operation.

My surgeon told me to use crutches for three months and then a walking stick for another six weeks, but two days after the operation I was happily walking up the hospital corridor to the shower – no crutches, unassisted and without pain – only to be told off by my nurse!

After 10 days at home, receiving BodyTalk Access from my wife twice a day and with virtually no pain, I threw away my crutches and returned to renovating my boat. A month later, we embarked on a world trip (not on the boat), which included lots of walking and climbing – all done with no pain!

BodyTalk has made me realize the amazing ability of our bodies to self-heal – trauma, emotions, illness, physical injuries, etc. – enabling us to enjoy life to the full. At 73, I now look forward to a more enjoyable third age!

Midwifery

Midwifery is a rapidly expanding area of BodyTalk. We have obstetrician/gynecologists who are BodyTalkers and have had their midwives trained in the BodyTalk System. In the cases in which they have used BodyTalk, we have seen a dramatic difference in the whole birthing process.

We know of one midwife who said that in the five years prior to her being trained in BodyTalk, her average deliveries were taking six to eight hours. After she was trained in BodyTalk and used simple techniques such as BodyTalk Access on her patients, the average time of delivery dropped to 60 to 80 minutes. This is a huge difference.

She also said that, when using BodyTalk Access, she is finding that the cervix dilates easier, the perineum relaxes, the back does not present as much of a problem and the contractions become regular far more quickly, In other words, the whole process is greatly enhanced by simply using these techniques. To make things even easier, the basic techniques of Access could be taught to the father so he could be doing them on the mother while the midwife takes care of her normal business – a huge boon. Plus, in the recovery stages, Access can be used to help the mother return to her normal, stable body rhythms, helping to ward off post-delivery emotional and stress factors.

The use of BodyTalk also can assist in breast feeding, if there is a problem producing milk. Very often, a mother's difficulties feeding her child breast milk are related to stress factors, almost like a post-traumatic stress disorder from child birth, and this can even lead to states of depression and many other unwanted symptoms. However, using BodyTalk on the mother over the first few weeks after delivery will greatly facilitate recovery and increase her enjoyment of motherhood.

Infants

Another aspect of this is that BodyTalk Access can be used on babies, even newborns. We have found that if a baby is crying a great deal or having a lot of problems with wind, etc., these often are symptoms of stress. Luckily, infants tend to respond very well to the BodyTalk Access system. It is totally non-invasive and very gentle. There is absolutely no danger in using it; however, it can be a wonderful tool in helping parents cope with a new baby and allowing them to help their baby settle down, sleep better, digest its food with far fewer feeding problems and so on.

Therefore, BodyTalk Access is a must not only for mid-wifery but also for the parents of newborn children to use on themselves and their babies.

Education

Education is an area of particular interest for me as a father of four – two of whom have degrees in education and are heavily involved in education issues. My own experiences of using the Cortices and basic Access techniques in the educational setting are quite extraordinary.

We have seen groups of children who have major attention and behavioral problems and are very disruptive in class. Once we trained them to tap out each other's Cortices at the beginning of the day, however, there was a dramatic difference in their behavior, their learning curve, their ability to read and their desire to learn.

Their teachers, of course, were quite stunned by the results.

Attention and behavior problems are a major issue in education these days, due to the high levels of stress on students and teachers in classrooms around the world. Therefore, we need a system that becomes a school routine at the beginning of the day – and even at the end of the day – in which children simply tap out each other's Cortices.

During the initial training, we have found there are a lot of giggles and embarrassment about doing something that is a little strange to them. However, our experience is that once the students have done it for about a week, they are very keen to continue and, in fact, often ask if they can tap each other's Cortices after lunch because they have found such a difference in the way they feel.

This training has proven to be very successful, and we have taught Access in various countries throughout the world in classroom situations with the children and their teachers learning to use it on themselves and each other. We have many cases in which we have been told about children who have then gone home and used it on their parents and seen a huge difference in the way their parents behaved. This, of course, is quite fun for a 6-year-old who can go home and "treat" his Mum and Dad and see a difference in their stress levels.

This aspect of education pertains not just to young children. It also is beneficial right through to the post-graduate level because of the extraordinary stresses on high school and university students to excel. Access could provide them with the ability to settle down before an exam, avoiding that state of mild "exam shock" that keeps so many students from performing well.

We have found that students who tap themselves out just before they go into an exam show a dramatic improvement in their performance and their grade. That is because BodyTalk helps to reduce their anxiety and stop what we call the switching factor, a phenomenon in which they can get their answers jumbled and mixed up, giving the wrong answers even though they know the correct ones.

A major goal of the International BodyTalk Foundation (IBF) is to have Access taught in as many schools as possible throughout the world, greatly improving education systems and, of course, contributing to the general health and well-being of the students and teachers involved.

Prisons

Obviously there are very few places in the world where you will see more stress than in a prison. And the sad thing is that so many of the people who are in prison are there because they were sick in the first place.

For many, the wiring in their brains had been badly damaged, probably due to high stress in fetal life and a high-stress upbringing that resulted in the hijacking of the brain by the amygdala, which I discussed earlier. This very often can lead to criminal behavior, and it certainly leads to all the anxiety, fear and then rage demonstrated by so many criminals.

I look forward to a time when we begin to realize that, in the majority of cases, so-called criminals are often people who are sick; they have disruptions in the functioning of their brains that can be treated effectively – just like addictions and many other mental disorders. I also look forward to a time where we start treating criminals proactively rather than just locking them up into a system that trains them to be more hardened criminals and increases their likelihood of maintaining a criminal lifestyle when they leave.

I feel strongly that if Access techniques were taught in prisons, the prisoners would utilize them because the majority of them do want to improve their quality of life, do want to feel better, do want to maintain their health. They also would appreciate something that calmed the volcano inside them – the internal anger or distorted way of thinking that makes their lives a misery and causes them to maintain a criminal lifestyle.

The process would be a very cheap one to effect, and it even could be set up for prisoners to treat each other. The changes, I am certain, would be dramatic, not only in the health and behavior of individual prisoners while in prison, but also in the overall amount of tension and violence in such institutions. Most importantly, perhaps, it would improve the prisoners' ability to go through rehabilitation and be restored as constructive members of society.

Corporate World

Access could have huge benefits in corporate life. Obviously the first aspect of the corporate world is that you treat any company like a community. Therefore, if Access is not available in the home or in the neighborhood, then what better place to introduce it than in the workplace?

There are many reasons to introduce Access into the corporate setting.

On the humanitarian level, the training of people to use Access techniques on one another at the beginning of the work day will help them maintain their health, reduce their stress levels, improve their brain function, focus better and, therefore, be far more productive and happy.

Of course, the other factor from a corporate point of view is the bottom line. A major pressure on profits is the lack of productivity due to stress, that is, the number of sick days and personal days that are taken. It also costs companies a great deal of time to correct mistakes made by people who are stressed out (what we call switched) or who are in a constant state of fight-flight under their work conditions.

I feel very strongly that any company that gave its staff the one-day training in Access for use on themselves and their families would see a significant improvement in bottom-line profits. This is because Access can help workers enjoy their work more, massively increase productivity, decrease their stress and reduce the need for sick days. Also important is the public relations aspect of taking a hands-on approach to helping staff members to feel better and realize that the business is doing something proactive to maintain and improve their lifestyle and health.

Developing Countries

Healthcare in developing countries is a key area of concern, because all the situations seen in Western society are often multiplied in underdeveloped nations.

Children learning Access techniques in Zambia, Africa.

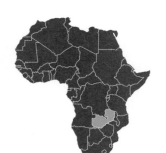

There is a severe lack of medical facilities in so many Third World countries, and the standard of health care is very poor to start with. Right now, because of huge populations and low taxation income, the average government cannot afford to supply the so-called high-tech Western approach to healthcare. So bringing in a basic hands-on approach such as BodyTalk Access, which can be done within communities and villages, is going to save the governments millions and millions of dollars per year and at the same time greatly improve the quality of life of their people.

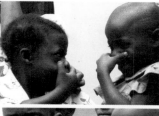

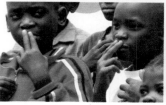

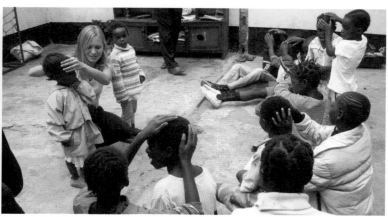

Our own experiences in teaching Access in villages in places such as India, Africa and South America have proved what a dramatic difference it can make. The villagers love it and take to it very easily because of the nature of it – it is energy medicine. They are very sensitive to it. They feel the changes immediately, and they do the work with a great deal of enthusiasm. The wonderful thing about Access is that it can be taught to them even if they are illiterate and have no education, because the techniques are so simple. We have found that indigenous people very quickly learn them, use them constantly and take advantage of them. This is a very exciting field for us. We just need funding so we can get more and more people out into the field to teach Access in these very remote and rural areas or even in the poor areas of cities so that everybody can start reaping the tremendous benefits of the BodyTalk Access program.

Sports and Performance

There are two aspects to the use of BodyTalk in sports and other physical performance activities.

We already have discussed the first, which is the treatment and rehabilitation of injuries, in which BodyTalk and even Access can play a huge role. The other aspect, however, is the utilization of the BodyTalk System to maximize the health of the sports person or performer, and in doing so, maximize his or her ability to compete.

Field Hockey

Taryn Edge, CBI - Durban, South Africa

I was at my 14-year-old daughter's indoor hockey match, the last one of the season. The team and I were sitting high up in the stands, overlooking the match under way. "Girls, do you wanna win this match?" I asked. "Yes," they responded. "Well then, pair up," I instructed; "we're gonna do some BodyTalk Access on each other to improve your concentration, coordination, energy levels, etc."

We did Cortices, Switching and Reciprocals. After we had finished, the girls were amazed at how relaxed and calm they felt and how energized they were. One of the girls commented that she felt like she could run a marathon.

Making goal after goal, they won 8-2 – the first victory of the whole season!! It was awesome to see. They were all on such a high as they ran out of the arena, "This BodyTalk must work!" one girl shouted. Another said, "I've never scored a goal in my life."

The coach actually came up to me after the match and said, "I just want to thank you for what you did with the girls. I've never seen them this lively on the court before." He hadn't a clue what we'd done; he had just seen this bunch up above tapping away.

"It's BodyTalk," I told him, "and I can come and teach it at the school, to you and the other sports coaches, so that you can do it with the girls before each match next year." He sounded very keen.

Athletes who utilize BodyTalk Access tell us that if they use it just before a game or before they compete, they seem to have a much more clearly functioning brain, their coordination and ability to go into "zones" is improved, their stress levels drop and, thus, their performance is improved. We have seen this in marathon runners and sprinters, in basketball and baseball players, and so on. BodyTalk has been utilized by many of the world's elite athletes and sports personalities, and, by having Access just before they compete and after they compete for recovery, they are able to maximize the functioning of their bodies and the results they get without resorting to illegal drugs.

So this is a very exciting part of Access.

Of course, we are not just talking about elite or professional athletes, as we have used Access on children's teams such as school hockey and soccer squads. Whenever we have treated a whole team before a match, the coach has noticed a dramatic difference in the way the children played, the way they worked better as a team and, of course, the results they got. So this is a very exciting field, which can be part of any sports program from youth leagues to the Olympic level.

Access has also shown terrific results when individual performers such as dancers and gymnasts have utilized the Access techniques before their competitions. The increased mental focus and tuned-in coordination of mental and physical balance that result from a brief Access session allow competitors to attain their personal best performances.

Dancing

Tracey Worrall, CBP - Brantford, Ontario, Canada

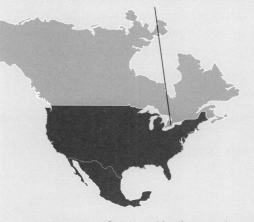

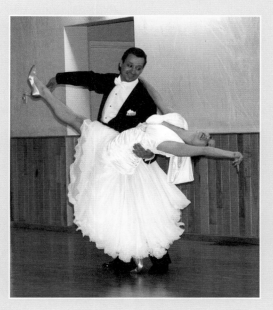

I am a professional ballroom dancer and Certified BodyTalk Practitioner. At a recent dance competition, my husband (an Access Technician) and I decided to put the Access techniques to the test. My husband was competing with a few of our young female students. The first round of competition was a bit rough for our students, definitely not their best performance. While standing in the "on deck" area waiting for the next round, we decided to "tap out" our students, working our way through the Access protocol. Despite the fact that a few strange looks were directed our way, the girls were happy to

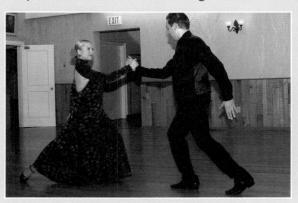

add a few new "steps" to their warm-up! The next round was amazing. Our students each performed at their personal best, and the results showed as they each won first place in their category! We are now working Access into our regular warm-up routine, not only for our students, but for our own performances.

Preventive Maintenance

Finally, let me reiterate that while BodyTalk Access is excellent to use in the treatment of stress and the improvement of health and the immune system and also can be used in crisis and first-aid therapy as a proactive way of addressing many symptoms and illnesses, we believe it is best used in preventive maintenance.

Cortices - More Than Just a Parlor Trick

Robert Burkwit - Venice, Florida, USA

After taking a day-long Access class, my wife and I went to a dinner party later that same night. We were explaining the Access class to our friends when I asked, "Does anyone have any pain?" One of the ladies at the table said she had had a headache that seemed to linger near the back of her neck for the last six months. She was taking six Advil a day at this point to help with the pain, but nothing seemed to work. I asked if I could show her the Cortices technique I had just learned earlier in the day. She agreed and afterwards her headache was completely gone, just like that! My wife, Mary, saw the lady three months later and asked her if the pain had come back. The lady said, "No, ever since then I have had no pain whatsoever."

In other words, by having people tap themselves out on a regular basis as a habit – like any other part of the daily routine – we are going to see significant changes in the quality of life, the clarity of the mind, the functioning of the immune system, the reduction of any addictive behavior patterns, and the prevention of disease and injury . This is because the person will be operating at much lower stress levels and with far better functioning of the immune system, which means they are not going to get sick as often.

This is a very important aspect of healthcare, and Access is one of the few techniques available that has excellent results and yet is simple to do and takes only a few minutes a day.

AnimalTalk Access

As I mentioned in an earlier chapter, BodyTalk works wonderfully with animals. Animals are generally more in touch with their instincts and their body's natural ability to heal itself. And there is generally less emotional clutter to interfere with these natural processes. So their receptivity to the energetic signals of a BodyTalk session is not hindered; and the results show it.

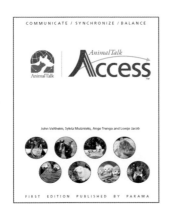

The AnimalTalk Access training manual currenly is translated and taught in English and German.

There is an advanced module in the BodyTalk curriculum for those who work with animals professionally. Veterinarians and trainers around the world are finding how BodyTalk can enhance their work. In a similar approach to BodyTalk Access for humans, we have developed AnimalTalk Access for laypeople to use on their own pets and companion animals. The results have been terrific. With only slight differences to the human Access technique routine, AnimalTalk Access can be used to alleviate minor pains and sicknesses that our animals are prone to, and can strengthen their general health and well being.

Access in Pre-Op on a Pony

Trishia van der Nest - Johannesburg, South Africa

Beanie, a Nooitgedacht pony, became pregnant in September 2005. All went well until June 2006 – when she appeared to have a prolapsed abdomen. Our local vet wasn't able to help us and suggested we send her to a larger facility. There, she was diagnosed with a ruptured hernia in her abdomen, through which part of her uterus was protruding.

The vets managed to induce labour and pull the foal out, as Beanie was unable to push her out. After the foal, Jelly Bean, was born – the vets' main aim was to keep Beanie alive, in order to get the foal on her feet and old enough to survive without her mother. The prognosis was very negative, and they all agreed that we should consider euthanasia for Beanie. They informed us that they could do a hernia repair operation, but these seldom worked in horses due to the tremendous weight bearing down on the repair.

At this stage, while driving to visit Beanie one afternoon, I heard a talk on the radio about BodyTalk. That week I went to a talk by Dr. John Veltheim and followed this with a visit to a BodyTalk practitioner. Then I decided to take the BodyTalk Access class.

Soon after this, a vet arrived from the USA and indicated he would like to attempt the hernia repair on Beanie. We were told again that the chances of success were not good. The repair operation was carried out some weeks later, and I visited Beanie the day following the surgery.

I used the five Access techniques I had learned on Beanie – I tapped her as I would have a person. The vets were amazed at Beanie's progress. She stood up fairly soon after the operation (which is unusual) and has continued to go from strength to strength. The veterinary hospital now cites Beanie as their "miracle case."

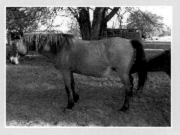

Beanie now is back at our farm with her foal, Jelly Bean, and both are thriving. Beanie runs, bucks, kicks and rolls, and the repair has remained fully intact, with no problems.

Beanie is seen here nursing with Jelly Bean

Animal Talk Fast Aid

Loesje Jacob, CBI – Armstrong, British Columbia, Canada

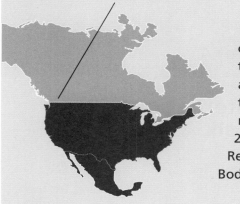

I was teaching an 'Obedience in the Bush' class for dogs. A Golden Retriever was barreling through the bush as only Goldens can. He ran into another dog and was screaming and writhing on the ground. When I got there I could tell he had really injured his hip. Fast Aid to the rescue. Within 20 minutes the Golden was up and 'barreling' again. Result…the vet taking my class is now a Certified BodyTalk Practitioner.

Ingested Antifreeze

Ange Trenga, CBI – Missoula, Montana, USA

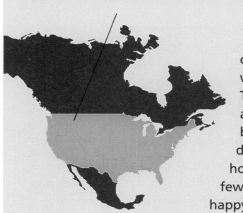

My Border Collie, Sparky, drank from a puddle of antifreeze late at night. We live in an area where emergency veterinary care is not available. Throughout the night, he would become lethargic and disoriented, with loud noises coming from his belly. After Access was applied, he would have diarrhea and then immediately perk up for several hours. AnimalTalk Access protocol was applied every few hours all night long. By morning, he was alert, happy and fully recovered from the poison.

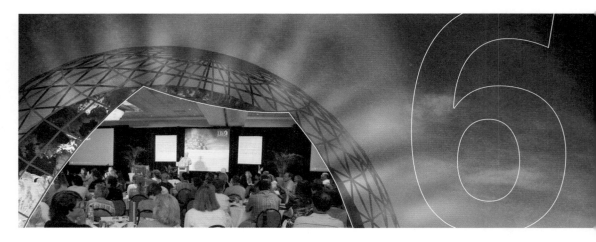

Chapter 6 The International BodyTalk Association

The International BodyTalk Association (IBA) is a world-wide organization providing vision, tools and training for the future of life science.

The IBA was formed in Sarasota, Florida, in 2000 by John and Esther Veltheim to be the official governing organization for the BodyTalk System and its ever-expanding suite of related modalities. The Association has some 3000 members in more than 30 countries and branch offices in Germany and Australia.

The IBA is responsible for the direction of BodyTalk and its family of life science systems; practitioner standards and credentialing; training and scheduling of courses, and generally working to ensure that the public's best interests are being served with regard to the practice and instruction of BodyTalk.

The IBA has more than 100 certified Instructors and Trainers teaching its various curricula. The training regimen for instructors is rigorous, and the certification standards are high in order to ensure that these powerful modalities are taught at the highest professional level possible.

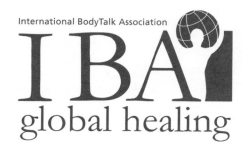

International BodyTalk Association

IBA

global healing

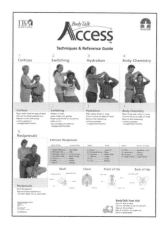

Access Manual poster available for reference once the class has been taken.

Our Web site, www.ibaglobalhealing.com, lists the professionally accredited BodyTalk practitioners in all the countries in which BodyTalk is practiced. Persons interested in advanced BodyTalk sessions should not go to anyone who is not on that list. This does not apply to BodyTalk Access, as Access does not require a professional qualification for use.

The IBA also supplies textbooks, promotional literature, videos and other materials for its Members, all of which can be purchased on the IBA Web site. Our books and many of our DVDs, CDs, booklets and IBA apparel also are available to the public.

As Access is just a fraction of the overall BodyTalk System, healthcare professionals and lay persons who want to be able to address a wide range of health challenges should visit our Web site to see how BodyTalk can be utilized in just about every facet of health care.

And anyone interested in any aspect of BodyTalk should visit www.ibaglobalhealing.com regularly, to keep up on the news and the growth of this amazing wellness system.

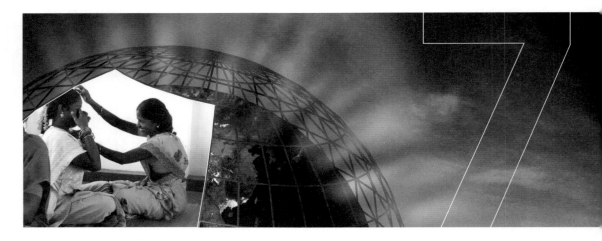

Chapter 7   The International BodyTalk Foundation

The International BodyTalk Foundation (IBF) was established as a 501(c)(3) non-profit organization under the U.S. Internal Revenue Code. Its primary objective is research and education in the BodyTalk System.

The IBF fulfills its mission through two branches of programs. The first branch involves promoting independent scientific studies that can demonstrate and document the efficacy of the BodyTalk System as an effective healthcare and health maintenance modality.

The second branch of IBF programs is designed to fund outreach projects for bringing BodyTalk Access to less fortunate neighborhoods and regions around the world where access to basic affordable healthcare is limited.

The IBF and Access

By teaching the very simple Access program to local groups, we are able to encourage them to take responsibility for much of their basic healthcare. In this way, we save the communities and countries a great deal of money, which can then be channeled into the higher-level healthcare systems for more serious medical conditions.

Donations to the IBF

In many of the communities to which we travel to teach BodyTalk Access, the people are unable to pay for the training. In those cases, the IBF helps to sponsor their training, manuals and the costs for the instructors to travel there.

Eventually, our goal in each area is to train some of the local people to become Access Trainers themselves, so the community can become self sufficient. At the time of this writing, programs such as this are already under way in several African countries, in India and in South America.

Those who wish to play a role in this outreach can contribute in many ways – from providing monetary support to volunteering their time, from helping us get the message out to providing their expertise to further our efforts. If you cannot provide such assistance yourself, perhaps you know someone who can. The more people we can get involved in, and behind, this effort, the healthier our world can be.

The IBF has an objective that is very similar to the old Chinese proverb that says: "Give a man a fish and you feed him for a day. Teach a man to fish and you feed him for a lifetime."

BodyTalk Access provides a powerful tool that can enhance both life and self-sufficiency, empowering people to take care of a great deal of the healthcare needs of their families or communities – gradually increasing the groups' total well-being and overall quality of life.

If you would like to be part of this vision, we urge you to visit our Web site, www.bodytalkfoundation.org There you will be able to find more information about IBF programs and plans, and you will see the many ways in which you can support the IBF in this critical healthcare mission.

If only every global challenge could be alleviated as simply!

Australia Austria Bahamas Belgium Botswana

Brazil Canada Cayman Islands Denmark Germany

Honduras Hong Kong India Indonesia Italy Japan

Kenya Malta Mexico Namibia Netherlands New

Zealand Poland Singapore South Africa Spain

Sweden Switzerland Taiwan United Kingdom

United States Zambia Zimbabwe

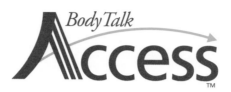

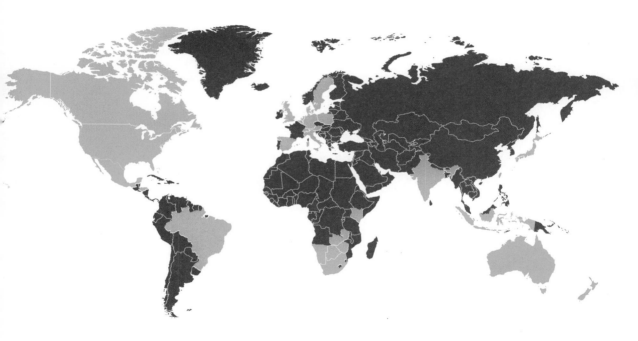

As of early 2008, BodyTalk Access has been taught in
33 countries around the globe.

Photo Credits:

Special Thanks to: Karen Fair, Janet Galipo, Renata Pilnik, Beverly Lutz, Katrin Bergstrome, Rosilyn Kinnersley, Debbie Zacharias, Taryn Edge, Sharon Gelber, Karen Atkins, Brett Selby, Loesje Jacob, Charlotte Nielson, Phillippa Peddie, Karla Kadlec, Lauren Brim, Tracey Worrall, Trishia van der Nest

Also Many Thanks to Cliff Berry for Graphic Design and Bonnie Limbach for Editing